Portion Perfection
International Edition
A visual weight control plan

First published 2014. Australian edition first published 2008.
© Great Ideas in Nutrition 2014, Phone +61 7 55366400, Australia

All rights reserved. No part of this book may be reproduced or transmitted in any form by any means, electronic or mechanical, including photocopying, recording or by any information storage or retrieval system, without prior permission in writing from the author.

The views expressed herein are those of the author and not necessarily those of the publisher or editor. This book is sold on the understanding that it is intended as a guide to educate and motivate but is not intended to replace professional advice.

Author: Clark, Amanda, 1964-

Title: Portion Perfection International Edition: A visual weight control plan / Amanda Clark.

Edition: 1st Ed.

ISBN: 978-0-9925043-3-5

Subjects: Cookery. Low-fat diet-Recipes. Health. Nutrition.

Dewey Number: 641.563

Editor: Melissa Groves

Design: Simone Young – www.tweedcoastgraphicdesign.com.au

Photography: Brett Backhouse and Enigma Visions

Food Styling: Lloyd Hanger

Nutrition Assistants: Anna Millichamp, Belinda Martin

Printed by Classic Offset Pte Ltd, Singapore

Disclaimers

While all care has been taken in the preparation of this book and every effort has been made to represent product details correctly, no responsibility is accepted for any errors, omissions or inaccuracies, or for any representation whether expressed or implied, which is beyond the control of the author/publisher. Foods represented in this book are as per generally available brands. Some estimates have been made.

Not every food that meets the criteria appears in this book and it would not be practical/feasible to do so. The book is intended as a guide rather than an exhaustive listing of all products which meet the criteria. The appearance of a product in the book is at the discretion of the author and is not guaranteed even if it meets all criteria. No fee has been paid/received in return for any reference to a product in the book.

Further, the criteria for inclusion/determination of everyday or occasional foods have been set with reference to various sources of existing criteria and the author's own professional judgment. Criteria may change based on current nutritional knowledge or research. Glycemic index (GI) is considered to be an important factor in selecting appropriate products for weight control. Not all products have been measured for GI. Therefore some professional discretion has been exercised based on the author's experience and no correspondence will be entered into.

Calories shown may be approximations and rounded to the nearest 100 Calories for ease of calculations. Also, breakfast cereal volumes have been rounded to the nearest ¼ cup. Protein contents have been rounded to the nearest gram.

This book is intended to be used as a general reference. It is a general guide only and does not constitute advice on individual or particular circumstances, or a substitute for the advice of a health care professional on any specific health issue/condition. It is recommended that a dietitian or health care professional be consulted to check that a weight loss plan is suitable and that specific advice be sought in relation to any specific health issues/conditions. The author/publisher accepts no responsibility for any failure to seek or follow the advice of a health care professional and will not be liable for such failure. Every effort is made to represent products accurately. No responsibility is taken for errors or omissions.

Portion Perfection
International Edition
A visual weight control plan

by Amanda Clark Adv APD

Acknowledgements

A book often looks like it is by a single author, but a project such as this one has been the culmination of the efforts of many. I couldn't have done it without you.

My family: Ray, Aimon and Brodie Clark, and Jan and Ken Railton.

My staff and colleagues: Jenny Lahiff, Joanne Rackley, Kimberley Aalders, Laura Hosking, and Belinda Cullen.

My project team: Simone Young, Melissa Groves, Lloyd Hanger and Enigma Visions.

My mentors and experts: Allan Borushek, Rosemary Stanton, Catherine Saxelby, Garry Egger, Annette Sym, Peter Howard, Rick Kausman and George Blair West.

My international colleagues and with particular mention of Stacy Paine.

Finally to all my clients who have provided positive feedback on the things that worked and guidance on the things that didn't.

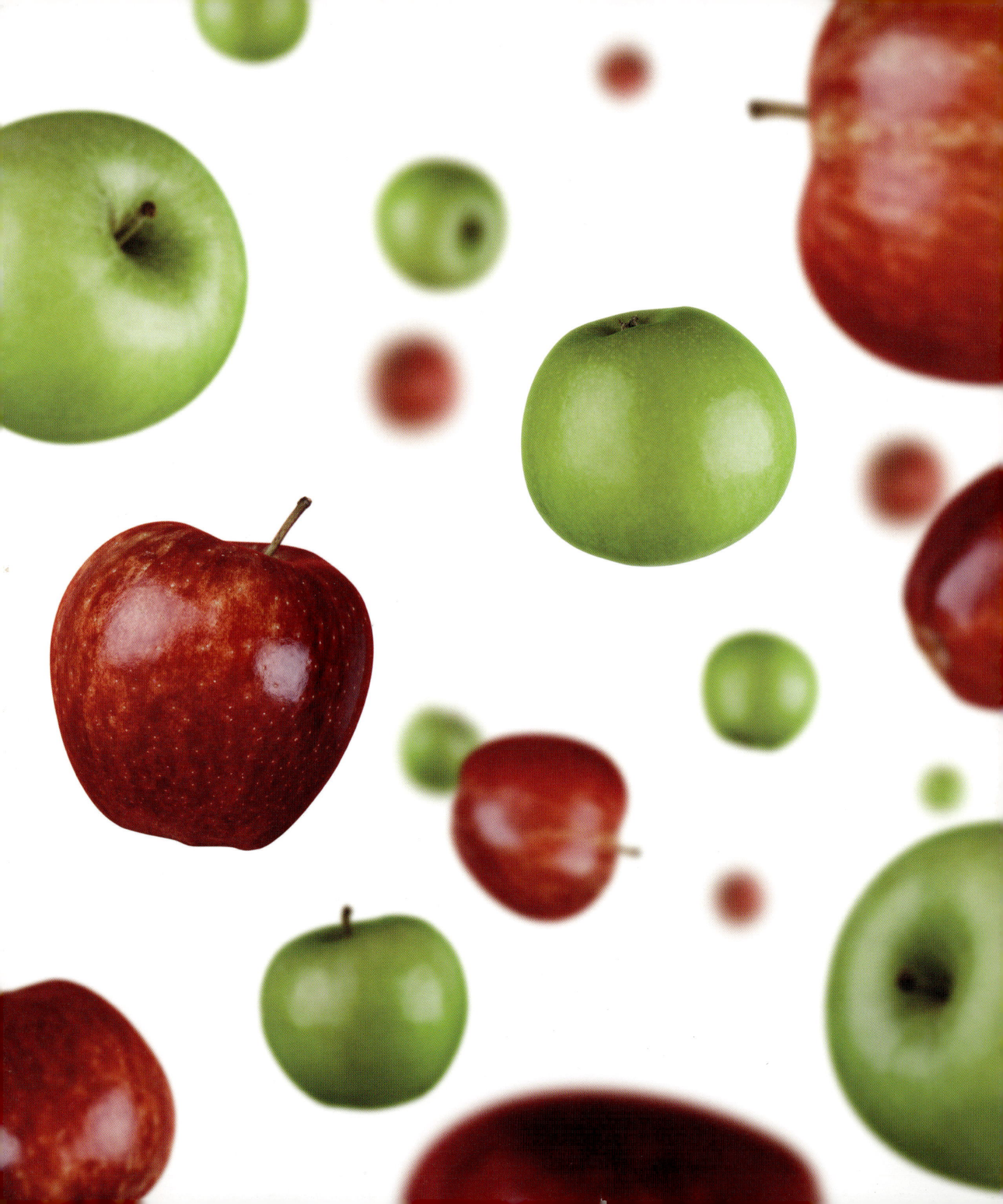

Foreword – by Allan Borushek

It is a pleasure for me to write the foreword to this unique book by Amanda Clark. She has over the years proven to be one of the most enterprising dietitians both in her clinical dietetic practice and in business (through her online nutrition resource shop).

Amanda has won several national awards for her innovative and practical approach and has gone on to be awarded Advanced status within the profession in Australia.

Now, Amanda has again shown her creativity by producing this book – a visual nutrition guide that provides practical information for the most effective use of her Portion Plate and Bowl.

Portion Perfection is the perfect guide for learning to control food portions. It will help you down-size to sensible portions and also show you how to improve the nutritional balance of your diet.

This educational resource is indeed timely in view of the global obesity epidemic which threatens to adversely affect the health of the nation through diet-related diseases such as type 2 diabetes, high blood pressure and heart disease.

Of great concern is that these diseases are occurring at increasingly younger ages – even as young as 10 to 12 years of age. The extra disease burden subsequently adds significant healthcare, economic and social costs to all nations. Indeed concerned governments from all developed nations are currently intent upon engaging the public in health initiatives that will hopefully tackle the obesity crisis.

What is clear is that most people need to be re-educated in the art of energy balance – the balancing of energy intake from food with energy output from physical activity. Over the years, we have adopted a lifestyle that is increasingly sedentary. At the same time, we are eating more food, which provides us with a net surplus energy intake – and a subsequent increase in body fatness.

It is no secret that oversized portions of food and drinks are contributing to this energy imbalance. Portion sizes have crept upwards over the last 20 years – and many common food products are double or triple their original size. It's been labelled 'portion distortion' and Amanda provides several examples in her introduction that will be recognised the world over.

The problem is that these overly large portions are treated as normal – particularly by children who have grown up with and expect to be served these standard large portions. Eating out presents its own set of problems, with some standard meals representing a whole day's worth of Calories; equally, some snacks and drinks can have the Calories of a whole meal.

Further, we are not good at estimating the weights or portion sizes of foods without the assistance of scales or measuring cups. Even experienced dietitians can have difficulty with such estimations.

All the above aspects are just some of the reasons why Amanda's Portion Plate and Bowls and accompanying book are such an important tool. They serve as self-monitoring tools to encourage healthy eating and weight control.

Amanda's book is highly innovative. It visually demonstrates precisely what different food portions actually look like. It takes the guesswork out of working out just what amounts of food comprise sensible portion sizes. The food photos add realism and colourfully demonstrate just how attractive and appetising well-balanced meals can be.

Amanda provides the tools to select healthier food choices and gives creative examples for healthy meals and snacks. Her easy-to-follow advice and professional expertise reflects her 25 years of clinical dietetic practice.

Any practical strategy that can break lifestyle or behavioural patterns that contribute to overweight or obesity – such as this book by Amanda – has to be applauded.

This book will also be welcomed as an instructional guide by dietitians as well as other health professionals and teachers involved with nutrition and dietetic education.

Here's to the perfect portion!

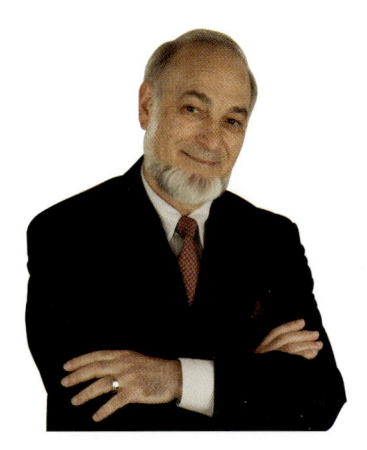

Allan Borushek
Dietitian & Health Educator
Member of the Dietitians Association of Australia

Contents

Introduction		10
Chapter 1:	Portion Problems Around the World	13
Chapter 2:	Introduction to the Tools and the Portion Perfection Concept	20
Chapter 3:	Nutritional Considerations	27
Chapter 4:	Portion Perfection in Practice	32
Chapter 5:	Food Guide Basics	38
Chapter 6:	Breakfasts	41
Chapter 7:	Snacks	63
Chapter 8:	Lunches	93
Chapter 9:	Dinners	110
Chapter 10:	Appendices	129

Introduction

In my 25 years of practise as a dietitian, one of my major priorities has been to make dietary concepts simple and understandable for my clients. I developed the Great Ideas in Nutrition Portion Perfection Plate for just that purpose. The Portion Perfection Plate is a dinner plate with ideal portion size and nutritional balance guides printed on it so that you can quickly and easily monitor the amount and type of food you serve. It also prompts you to slow down your eating to help you feel satisfied with smaller meal sizes. The Portion Perfection Bowl shows guides for cup amounts to help you serve the ideal amounts of cereals, soups and desserts. These products can be purchased online at www.portiondiet.com.

Expanding on that concept, the aim of this book is to help guide you through your food choices for the entire day. I've found that many people zone out when presented with a list of dietary options – but that they respond well to visual images, and so I often use pictures rather than words with my clients. *Portion Perfection* includes photographs of the ideal portion size for everyone in the family. Photos of actual foods have been used to enable you to recognise local brands and the nutritional criteria has been provided so you can check that the local version is healthy enough to eat every day.

It's easy to lose perspective when it comes to knowing how much to eat. Did you know that restaurant, take away and packaged food portions have been getting steadily bigger over the years? External factors like this certainly don't help us with our nutritional decision-making, and in this book I hope to give some answers to all those who have lost perspective when it comes to the question of *how much should I eat?*

Portion Perfection shows you the ideal portion sizings of common foods. This information will help you to decide whether to eat more or less of a particular meal or snack. Eating the right amount – and knowing the consequences of eating too much – will become truly simple.

I have found that the Portion Perfection concept helps both overeaters and undereaters, as well as those with serious eating disorders, and those just wishing to be more healthy and eat balanced meals.

I would also like to influence processed food manufacturers to take a look at the serving sizes that they offer the market. We are the customers, and if we let the market know that we want snacks in 100 Cal / 420 kJ serves then that is what we will get – eventually. Why not start the process at your local supermarket by choosing products that make it easy to eat a correctly portioned serve?

Portion Perfection will convince you that portion size is increasing, help you to figure out what your own dietary requirements are, and show you what your ideal portions actually look like. Seeing what the right serve looks like for either weight loss or weight maintenance really can help keep you on track. The plate and bowl concept is an effective way to monitor your progress on an ongoing basis, and can be used by the whole family.

This book is aimed at all adults, adolescents and children from five years of age aiming to achieve ideal body weight and maintain it. It's suitable for anyone in the family who is aiming to lose weight or hoping to avoid gaining weight.

Dietitians recommend an acceptable rate of weight loss to be anything between 2 pounds / 1kg per week and 2 pounds / 1kg per month for adults and teenagers over 13. Faster weight loss may result in fast weight regain, so is best avoided. For parents planning to use *Portion Perfection* with children younger than 13, we recommend that you consult with an Accredited Practising Dietitian (APD) to determine your child's individual Calorie and nutritional needs, as weight loss in childhood may prevent children from reaching their full growth potential. It is generally more appropriate to help children maintain their weight while they continue to grow, thereby getting leaner with age. I have provided guidelines for weight maintenance in overweight children here, however individual needs vary.

Recognising a Qualified Dietitian

In Australia, all dietitians who maintain their training to a high standard are APDs - this means they're Accredited Practising Dietitians. Some dietitians have been granted Advanced status. This identifies the top 1 per cent of the profession who are formally recognised as leaders in their field. In the UK dietitians must be registered with the Health Care Professions Council, and in the USA look for a Registered Dietitian.

I hope you find the book, plate and bowl useful so that you may turn your attention to other things in life and stop worrying about your weight. I welcome feedback on your experiences – please contact me via facebook at **www.facebook.com/portionperfection** or via the "Question" option on our homepage at **www.portiondiet.com**.

Amanda Clark

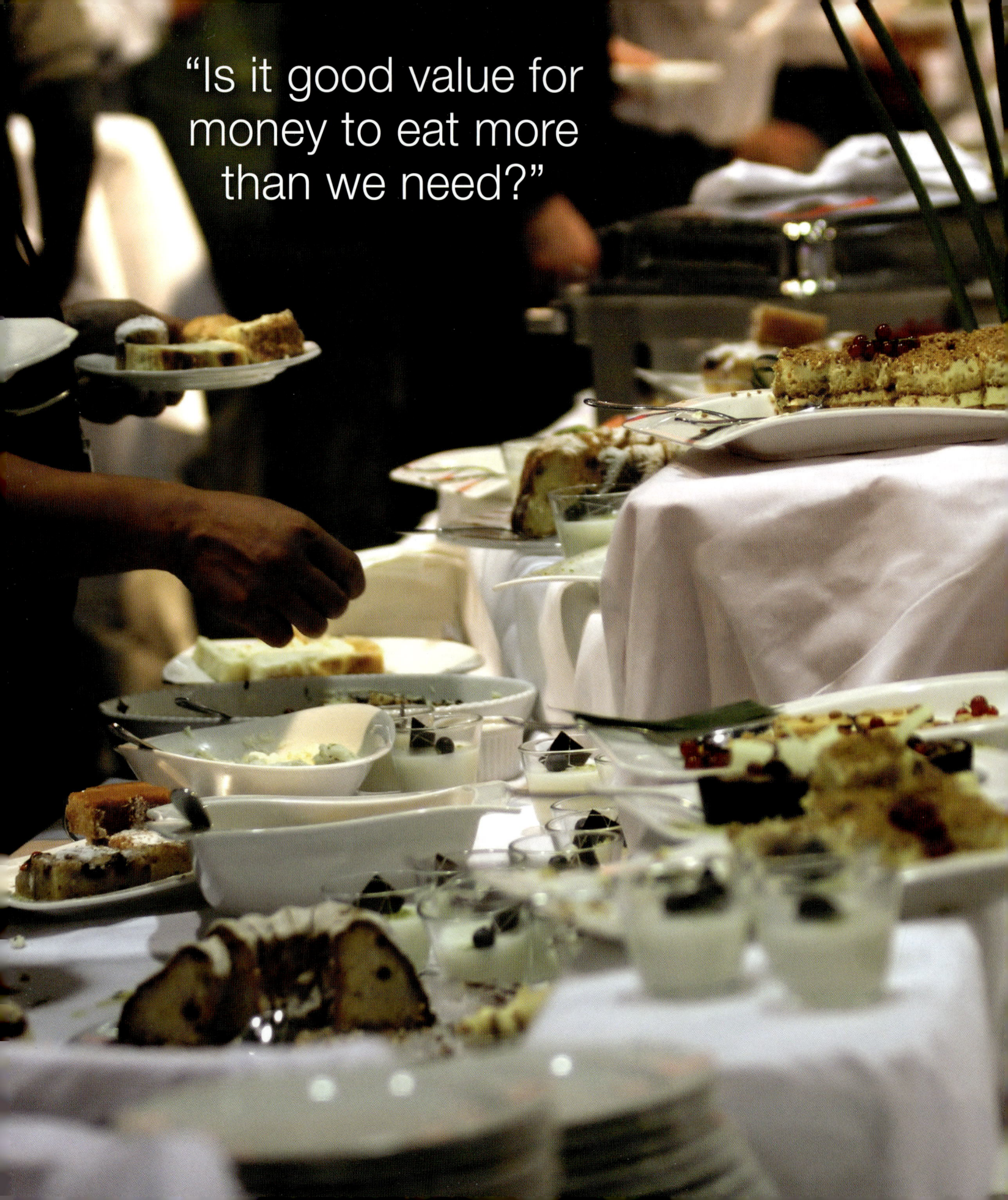

"Is it good value for money to eat more than we need?"

Chapter 1: Portion Problems Around the World

Recent data from Australia, the United States and Europe show that we are eating up to 500 Calories / 2100 kJ per day more than we did 20 or 30 years ago.

Experts agree that:

- We are eating more without being aware of it;
- Marketing encourages us to eat large serves of high-Calorie foods;
- Advertising encourages us to eat more often, and suggests that it's normal to eat occasional foods all the time, or at every meal.

It's also true that we generally do less exercise these days than we used to. And, of course, less exercise also contributes to the amount of food that we store as body fat.

The latest global estimates suggest that an additional 1,200,000,000 (1.2 billion) people will be overweight or obese by 2030, with the greatest proportion of those new qualifiers being residents of the UK, USA or Australia. The level of diabetes will likely follow and this is suspiciously in line with an ongoing increase in the Calorie content of many common food serves.

So many people are searching for the foods they can eat to sustain a healthy weight. Every year we're enticed by a new fad diet or the 'discovery' of a new diet secret or superfood. The more pertinent question, though, is to determine how much is the right amount of food to eat to *achieve and maintain a healthy weight.*

What we eat is certainly a problem for some, but *how much* we eat is becoming a problem for all of us.

In 2008, the Department of Human Services estimated that 73% of Australians will be overweight or obese by the year 2025.

We fear for the future of our children, and quite rightly so. The fact is that we have probably reached our maximum life expectancy potential, and even with the best medical care, our children may live shorter lives than we do.

Think Calories

We've shown both Calories and kilojoules in most areas of the book. Australia uses kilojoules as its proper metric measurement, but we find in practice that Calories are much smaller numbers, which are easier to add and multiply! So if you don't speak either language, start learning to think Calories to stay on track.
1 Calorie = approx 4.2 kJ, so roughly multiplying or dividing by 4 will convert Calories to kilojoules and vice versa.

What can be done to remedy the situation?

We all know that the level of obesity is rising among our family and friends. Rather than dwell on the statistics, let's focus on things that we can fix for ourselves.

First, let me introduce the concept of Calories (units of energy) in weight control. When we gain weight, what we are actually doing is eating more Calories than we are burning off. Our bodies then store away the excess as body fat.

So why are we consuming more Calories than we are burning off? The reasons are many and varied, and differ from person to person, but can include stress, lack of sleep, declining activity levels, busy lives, food marketing and increasing portion sizes. Other things like hormone imbalances can cause the signals your body sends you – for example, telling you that you need to eat more – to not function properly, so although you might have eaten enough, you don't feel satisfied.

Some of these things we have direct control over, and some we don't. While we wait for researchers to learn more about what might cause an imbalance in internal hormones, or hope that the food industry takes some responsibility for the way that food is presented to us, we CAN take some control over our levels of activity and the portion sizes that we eat.

Just as we haven't noticed that our portion sizes have increased, there is good evidence that we wouldn't notice if they decreased again – what a painless way to cut Calories!

So, let's look at re-establishing your knowledge about how much to eat.

> Overweight and obesity amongst adults have doubled over the past two decades. Such that the US, Mexico, New Zealand, Chile, Australia, Canada and the UK are now ranked as the fattest nations.
> **(OECD Obesity Update, 2012)**

What has happened to portion sizes?

I believe that clever marketing and eating too much have left us dazed and confused about how much we actually *need*. First, the facts, and then let's take a look at some Australian examples that I'm sure you can relate to at home.

A meal for weight maintenance ideally contains 450-550 Calories (Cals) / 1890-2310 Kilojoules (kJ), and a snack contains 200 Cals / 840 kJ.

Chocolate bars

Think back about 20 years ago, if you can! Can you remember how big chocolate bars were? Strangely, they were much smaller than they are today. For example, look at what's happened to the Kit Kat, which was one of the smallest bars on the market 20 years ago. Today, that very same snack is one of the largest on the market.

Originally Kit Kats were 0.7 oz / 20 g (around 100 Cals / 420 kJ), but now there's the Kit Kat Chunky King Size which is 2.75 oz / 78 g (409 Cals / 1717 kJ). It's gone from an acceptable snack to almost a meal's worth of Calories!

20 years ago:
100 Cals / 420 kJ
Today:
409 Cals / 1717 kJ

Let's look at some more comparisons between portion sizes 20 years ago and those today.

Take-away coffees

Twenty years ago, a take-away coffee would have come in a 7 fl oz / 200 ml polystyrofoam cup. It would have been made with water, and even if you added full cream milk and sugar, it wouldn't be more than about 85 Cals / 357 kJ.

Over the last fifteen or so years, though, there's been a coffee revolution. Where 20 years ago it wasn't that common to get a take-away – and many of us didn't even know what a latte was – now it's a different story. Think about the various different sizes of take-away cups, and all the milk-based coffees you can now order – lattes, flat whites and cappuccinos – and we start to see a problem. A regular milk-based coffee (and you can include hot chocolates here, too) would contain 200 Cals / 840 kJ. That's a 'Regular' but what about a 'Grande'? At 16.5 fl oz / 470 ml, a 'Grande' provides up to 480 Cals / 2016 kJ, depending on the particular drink you've ordered.

20 yrs ago:
85 Cals / 357 kJ
Today:
Up to 480 Cals / 2016 kJ

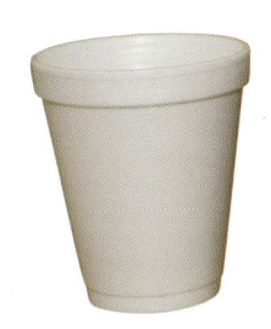

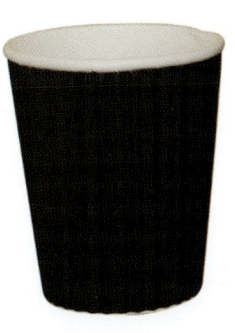

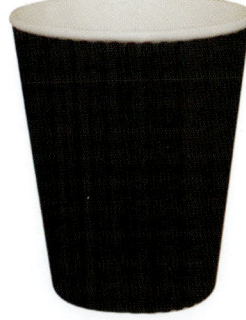

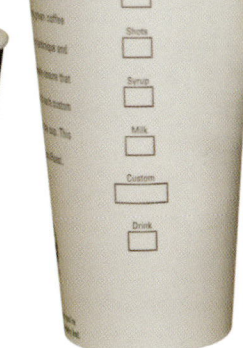

Flavoured milk

Twenty years ago, flavoured milk was sold in 10 fl oz / 300 ml cartons, containing 220 Cals / 924 kJ. Now 17-21 fl oz / 500-600 ml is more the norm, and the Calorie count is up to 440 Cals / 1848 kJ.

So a large milk drink doesn't go with lunch … it IS lunch!

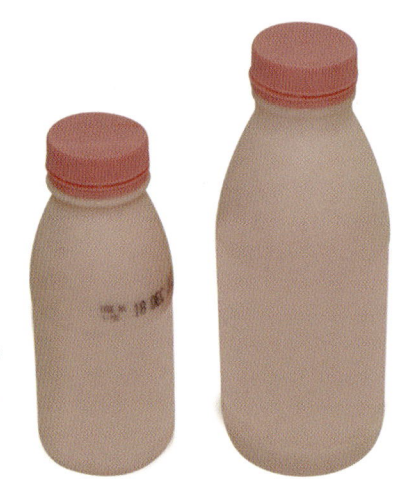

20 yrs ago:
220 Cals / 924 kJ
Today:
440 Cals / 1848 kJ

Chips / Crisps

Twenty years ago a packet of crisps weighed 1 oz / 30 g, today both 1.8 oz / 50 g and 3.5 oz / 100 g packets are marketed as single servings.

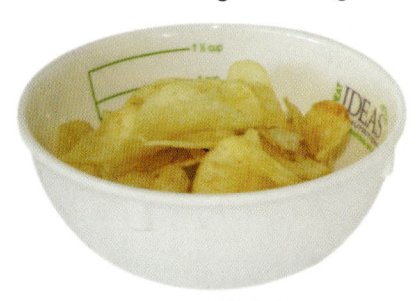

• 1 oz / 30 g = 150 Cals / 630 kJ

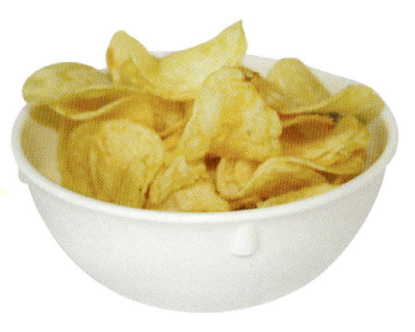

• 1.8 oz / 50 g = 250 Cals / 1050 kJ

20 yrs ago:
150 Cals / 630 kJ
Today:
Up to 500 Cals / 2100 kJ

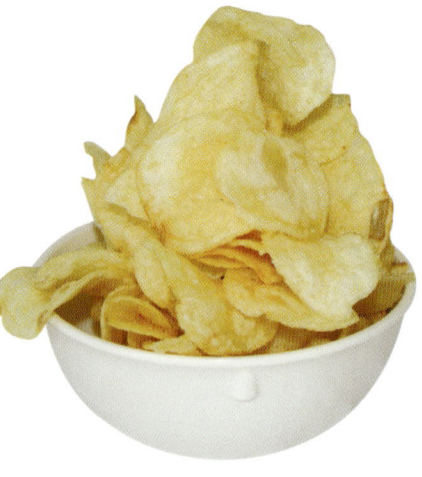

• 3.5 oz / 100 g = 500 Cals / 2100 kJ

Cookies

Twenty years ago a choc chip cookie contained 50 Cals / 210 kJ.

Today the jumbo cookies found in coffee shops can contain over 500 Cals / 2100 kJ.

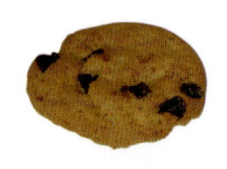

20 yrs ago: 50 Cals / 210 kJ
Today: 500 Cals / 2100 kJ

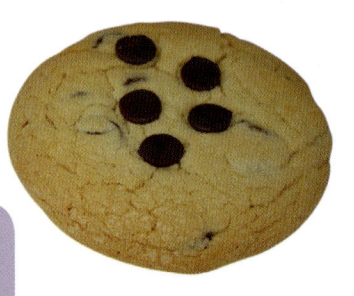

Sugary drinks

Now that manufacturers are pushing 21 fl oz / 600 ml bottles of sugary drink as the 'normal' size, the smaller size is starting to look like a cute, old-fashioned model.

- A 13 fl oz / 390 ml bottle contained 160 Cals / 672 kJ
  – okay for an occasional snack if you're a healthy weight.
- A 21 fl oz / 600 ml bottle contains 245 Cals / 1029 kJ
  – a hefty addition to any meal.

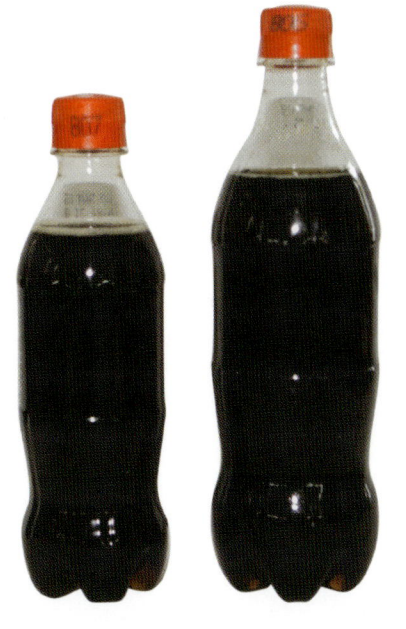

20 yrs ago: 160 Cals / 672 kJ
Today: 245 Cals / 1029 kJ

You may not have thought of drinks as snacks before. Calorie-containing drinks are a significant contributor to energy overconsumption Instead of thinking of it as 'just a drink', it's time to consider it as a food choice. If you're hungry choose something solid - not liquid.

Perfect Portions

So how did our portions get so big?

The main reason behind increasing portion size is simply that food manufacturers want to make more money, and they have a number of clever ways of achieving this.

Their aim is to persuade us to eat more of their products. There are two ways of doing this: they can sell more, although this isn't necessarily easy to do. The simpler option is to make the products bigger (and therefore more expensive).

Food is actually a fairly small component of the cost of a food product. The main costs are the labour, the packaging and the advertising. It is therefore a very cheap option to offer extra-large portions as an attractive offer to consumers. For example, you can get an upgrade on a take-away meal which gives you 50 per cent more food for 16 per cent more money. Or the company decides to manufacture a 'king-sized' packet, with a higher price, and then gradually phases out the original packaging size.

Another simple benefit of larger products from the manufacturer's point of view is: the bigger the packet, the more visible it is on the supermarket shelf.

Of course, consumers aren't entirely blameless, either. Where we fall down is that we are attracted to value for money deals – but is it good value for money to eat more than you need? What is the actual cost in health and efforts to lose that excess weight gained?

> **Value for money?**
>
> Our local donut franchise gives two free cinnamon donuts with every thickshake. For weight loss, the aim is 100 Calories / 420 kJ for a snack. The thickshake itself is equivalent to a large meal at 530 Cals / 2226 kJ – add the donuts and you're up over 1000 Cals / 4200 kJ!

Size matters

Many food packets have recommended serving sizes on the nutrition information panel. These can be very misleading.

For example, look at the label for this divine-sounding dessert. The heading at the top of the nutrition information panel says 'per serve', 470 kJ, which is only just over 100 Cals. This sounds appealing, right? But think again. The pack weighs 7 oz / 200 g – the same as a single-serve yoghurt tub – so it would be easy to think it is a serve. It's only when you study the label that you find that there are five servings per pack. One serve equals roughly one spoonful!

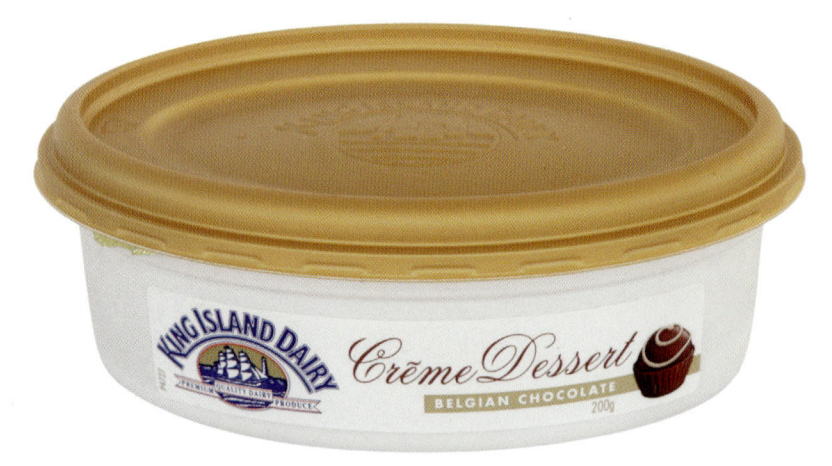

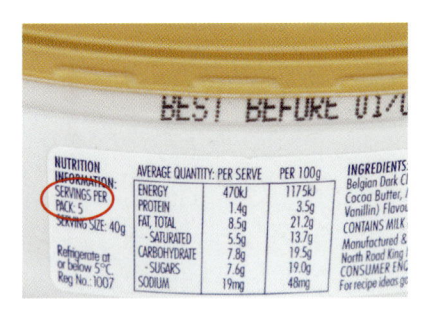

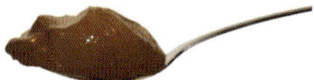

One serve equals roughly one spoonful!

"The larger the packet, the more we eat."

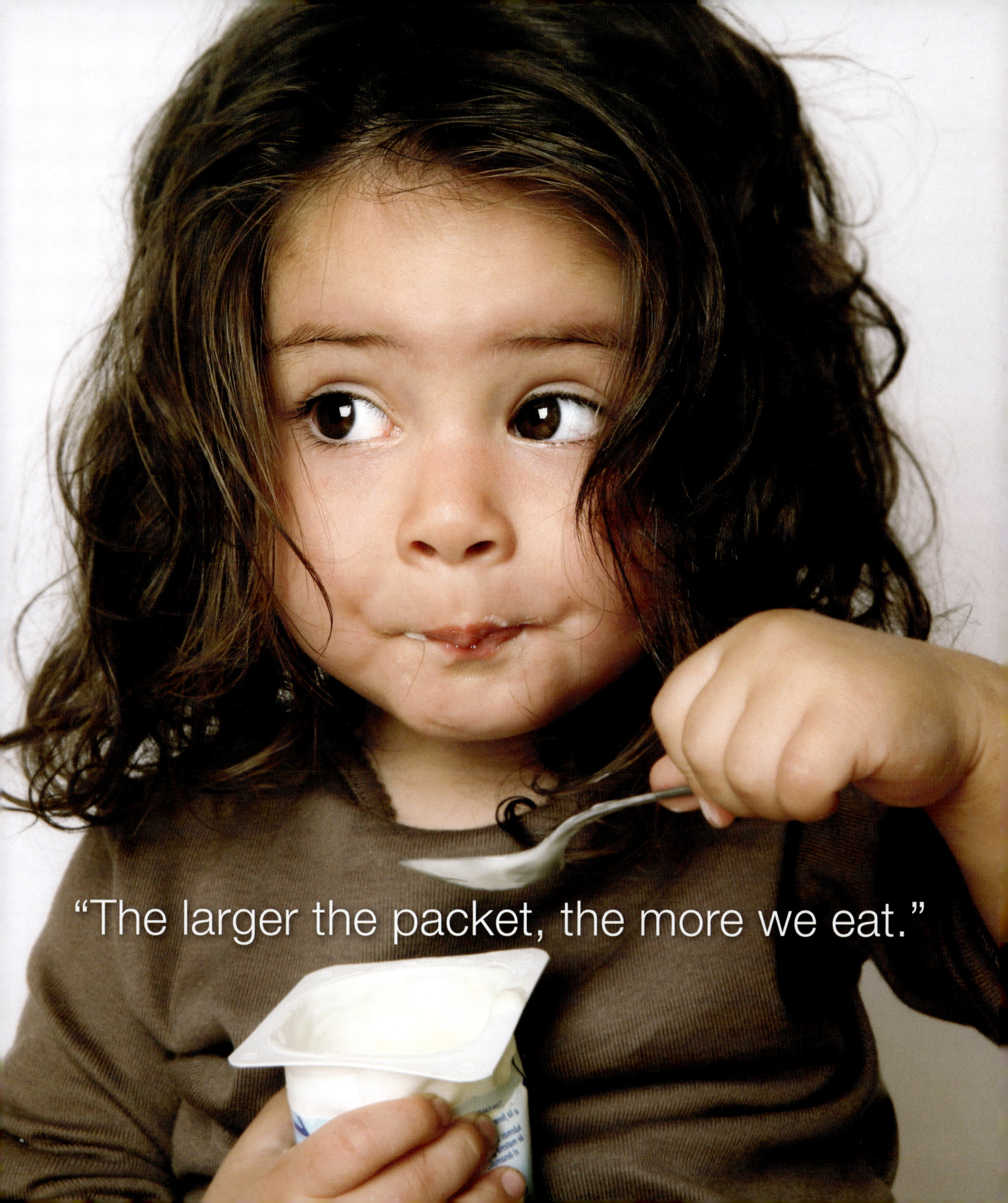

Chapter 2: Introducing the tools

The Great Ideas in Nutrition Portion Perfection Plates and Bowls serve as self-monitoring tools to help encourage healthy eating and weight control.

Melamine bowl

Melamine plate

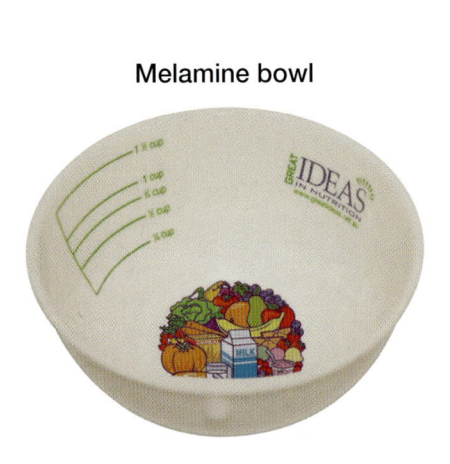

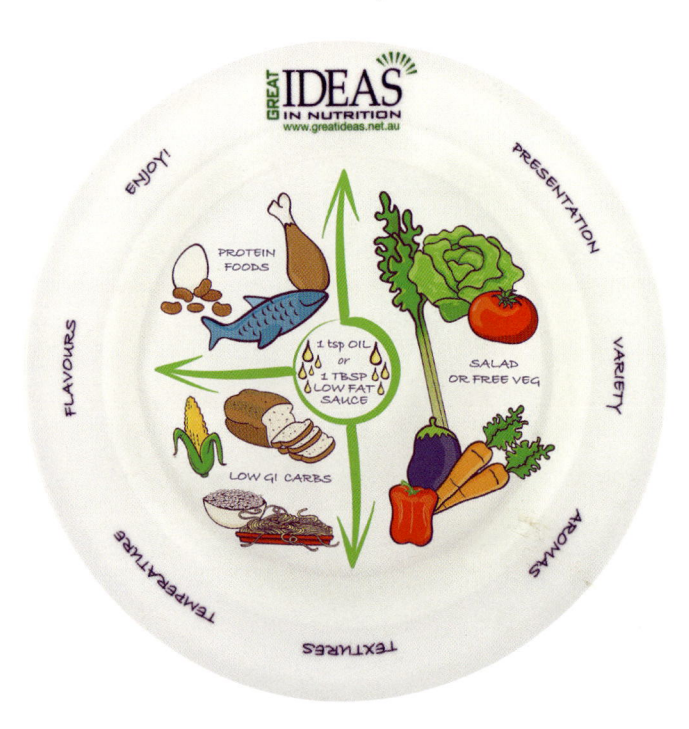

The tools address three common issues:

1. **Portion size**
   Whether you're trying to lose weight or just avoid gaining weight, portion control is a valuable tool.

2. **Nutritional balance**
   Getting the right things on your plate to get what you need is easy with the plate system.

3. **Eating awareness**
   By being fully aware of what you are eating, and eating in a 'conscious' way, you will find satisfaction for your mind as well as your stomach. This involves savouring your food and slowing down your eating so you feel satisfied with the smaller quantity.

Getting the right portion size

The plate is designed to hold 350 Calories / 1470 kJ when just the base is filled to a depth of ¾ inch / 2 cm in the middle, keeping the rim of the plate free of food.

When the melamine plate used in this book is filled to the edge, ¾ inch / 2 cm deep in the middle, it is approximately 450 Cals / 1890 kJ. Both melamine and porcelain versions are in production — check availability in your area at **www.portiondiet.com**. The rim of the porcelain plate is larger, so a series of green dots or sensory words on the plate's rim indicate the 450 Calorie / 1890 kJ boundary.

The section on page 32 entitled 'How much do I need?' enables you to work out your own personal plan and portion sizes.

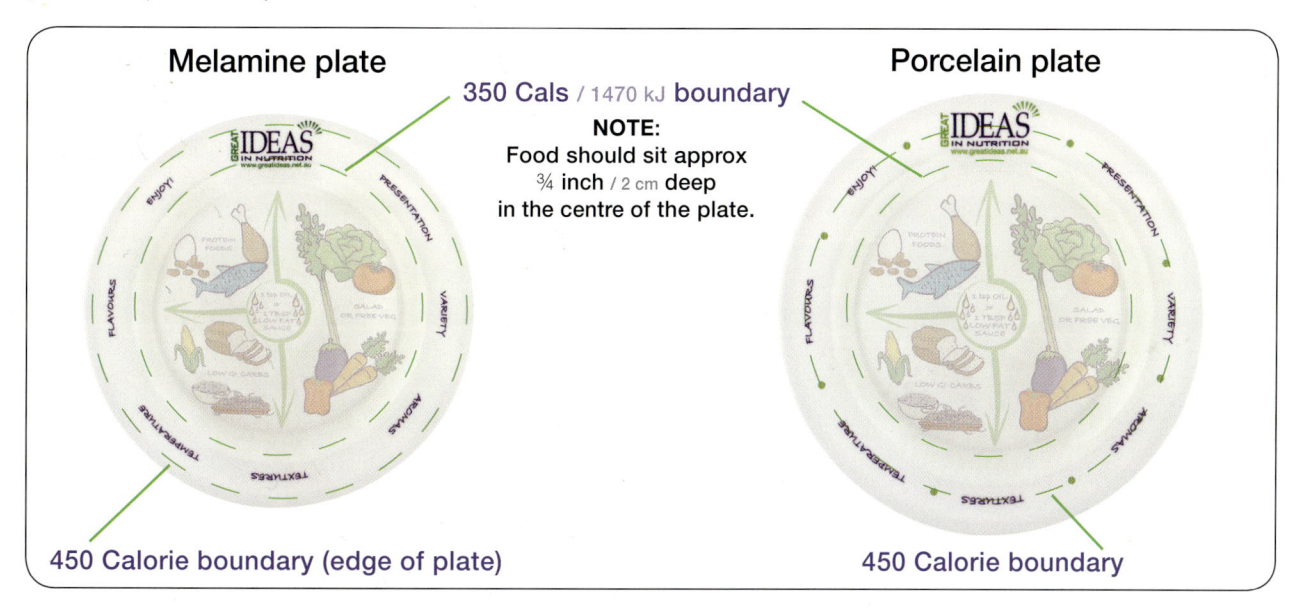

Melamine plate | **Porcelain plate**

350 Cals / 1470 kJ boundary

NOTE:
Food should sit approx
¾ inch / 2 cm deep
in the centre of the plate.

450 Calorie boundary (edge of plate) | 450 Calorie boundary

Finding nutritional balance

The Portion Perfection Plate is divided into segments that show the ideal proportion of protein foods to carbohydrate foods and vegetables for a balanced intake.

Many people are led to believe they need to avoid carbohydrates to lose weight. It's important not to be fooled into thinking we weren't designed to eat carbohydrates. That's what the enzymes in our stomach are for. Over half the world's population lives on carbohydrate-based foods as their staple – and most of those people don't have the obesity problem that we do in the Western world, so eliminating carbohydrates is not the answer.

Equally, there might be many other foods that you think you 'shouldn't eat' because they're not included in various popular diets. But with the Portion Perfection Plate, all you need to do is get the portion sizes right and you can enjoy all healthy foods – and some of the not so healthy ones – in the right quantities.

> **What does 'GI' mean?**
>
> The Glycemic Index (GI) is a rating system for carbohydrate foods, showing you how quickly each type of food raises your blood sugar levels. An example of a low GI food is grainy bread, whereas most white breads and pancakes are high GI foods.

We do know that protein is more satisfying than either carbohydrate or fat, so protein is encouraged in the form of dairy or soy products, meat or legumes.

The segments of the plate are to be filled by (see right):

- **Protein foods**: lean red meat, poultry, fish, egg, legumes (soy beans, baked beans, lentils, chickpeas, etc) or tofu.

- **Low GI carbohydrates**: sweet potato, peas, corn, basmati or doongara rice, pasta, rice noodles, grainy bread, a corn tortilla, couscous, quinoa, freekeh, bulgur, barley or spelt. This segment may also contain occasional amounts of baby potatoes, pita bread, parsnip, pumpkin, polenta or grits, which are all medium GI carbohydrates.

- **Salads and free veg**: alfalfa, artichoke, asparagus, bamboo shoots, bean sprouts, beetroot, broccoli, Brussels sprouts, cabbage, capsicum/peppers, eggplant, green beans, leek, lemon, lettuce, mushrooms, onions, radish, rhubarb, rocket, shallots, silverbeet, snow peas, spinach, spring onion, squash, sugar snap peas, swede/rutabaga, swiss chard, tomato, turnip, watercress, water chestnut or zucchini.

- **Low-fat sauces or dressings**: oil or oily dressings, commercial low-fat dressings or those based on fruit juice or low-fat mayonnaise, non fat milk sauces, low-fat gravy mixes, apple, honey-soy, oyster, mint, plum, BBQ, tomato, soy, hoisin, teriyaki, Worcestershire, chilli, sweet chilli, black bean or light (fat-reduced) cheese sauces.

> **What does 'free veg' mean?**
>
> Free veg is the term used for low-starch vegetables that have less than 20 Cals / 84 kJ in a standard serve and don't affect blood sugar levels. For example, tomato is a free veg, whereas potato is a higher-Calorie, starchy vegetable.

How to eat consciously

'Conscious eating' is a concept that comes from mindfulness psychology. It means eating with awareness, really looking at the food you intend to eat, smelling it, tasting it, savouring and enjoying it. This helps you reach satisfaction mentally as well as just filling the capacity of your stomach.

The words around the edge of the Portion Perfection Plate prompt you to consider the following every time you eat.

- **Presentation** – before you start eating, notice the way the food looks. Has it been served in an attractive manner? Does it look appealing? Pay full attention to the quantity that you see – this will help you anticipate when the meal has ended. This is a good reason never to eat from a multi-serve packet – always serve out the amount you intend to eat, or buy single portion-sized packs.

- **Variety** – do you see a variety of colours, textures and types of foods on your plate?

- **Aroma** – smell the food. What do you notice? Does it smell fresh? Appetising? Can you smell all the components of the meal, or only some?

- As you eat the food, notice the **texture** – is it smooth? Grainy? Tough? Tender?

- Also think about the **temperature** – is it ideal for that food? Could it be warmer or cooler?

- Savour the **flavours** – what ingredients can you taste? Imagine if you didn't see what you put in your mouth. Do you think you could identify it from the taste and texture?

- Slow yourself right down and **enjoy** the meal.

The Portion Perfection Bowl is available from the website and indicates cup amounts. This is a useful adjunct to the plate and appears in the program photos in this book.

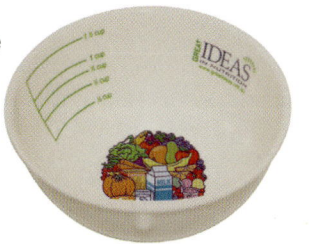

You can order online at: **www.portiondiet.com**

The value of portion control

There is much valuable research to show that the more food we put on our plates, the more we will eat. The scary thing is that we are not any more satisfied when we eat these larger portions.

In fact, the research shows that the larger the plate the more we eat; the larger the spoon the more we eat, the larger the packet or serving bowl the more we eat, the greater the variety offered, the more we eat. All without significant awareness.

You may think that you are too clever to be fooled by a larger bowl, but even nutrition experts get caught. One American study focused on 85 nutrition experts who were attending an ice cream celebration for a colleague. They were randomly given either a smaller (2 cup) or larger (4 cup capacity) bowl and either a 2 fl oz / 60 ml or 3 fl oz / 90 ml ice cream scoop. After serving themselves, their bowls were weighed while they completed a survey. This study found that even when nutrition experts were given a larger bowl, they served themselves 31 per cent more without being aware of it. They even served an additional 14 per cent if they used the larger serving spoon.

For more insight into the things we do, read *Mindless Eating* by Brian Wansink (available on our website at **www.portiondiet.com**).

Portion Perfection Plates and Bowls work!

Apart from my own experience, others around the world are testing out the same theory. A Canadian study published in the *Archives of Internal Medicine* in June 2007 showed that using a plate and bowl marked with portion sizes helped very overweight patients with diabetes lose weight. They were also able to reduce their use of medication to control blood glucose levels.

Case Studies

Melissa

Melissa is a teenager with a family history of weight problems. I found that Melissa's intake of high-Calorie snacks during and after school were a problem. By using the Portion Perfection photos for education rather than diet sheets or lists, Melissa can clearly recognise suitable snack choices. She is a potato crisp fan and she knows she can have them sometimes but finds when she's hungry she'd rather have a larger serve of fruit or yoghurt than one tiny packet of crisps. She chooses fruit because she wants to, not because she has been told to.

Fay

Fay is a middle-aged woman who has spent all her life feeling guilty about her eating. Our first step was to focus on conscious eating. Fay returned to her second consultation elated at the experience she had. She announced that the weight of guilt had lifted from her shoulders and she had tasted foods for the first time. She even noticed that some of the foods she'd clung to over the years didn't taste that great. She lost 4.5 lb / 2 kg in two weeks without any dietary instruction and this continued for some time before we needed to look more closely at portion size.

Brian

Bachelor Brian's eating habits were chaotic, with no structure and a poor intake of vegetables. His standard meal consisted of meat and eggs or potatoes. By using the Portion Perfection Plate, Brian gained a clear formula for planning an evening meal. He can now identify countless dinner combinations that result in the perfect meal.

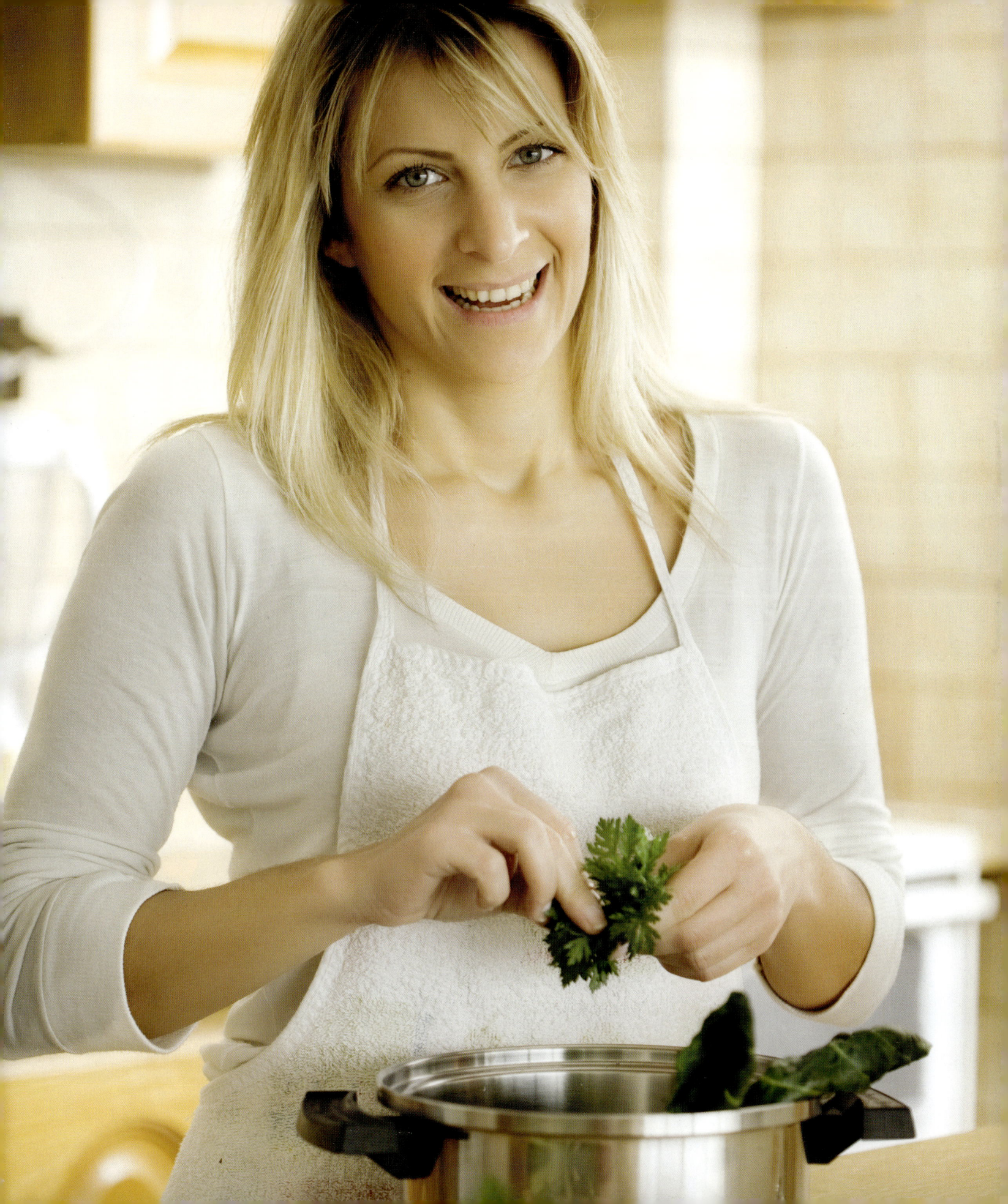

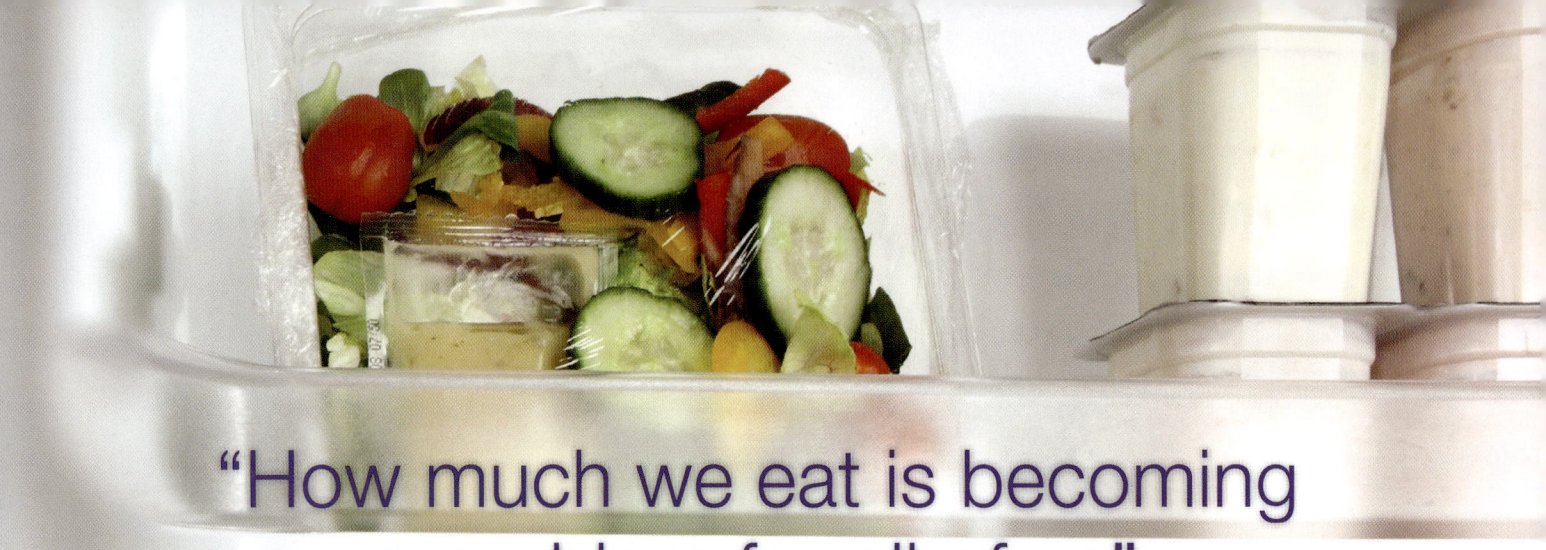

"How much we eat is becoming a problem for all of us"

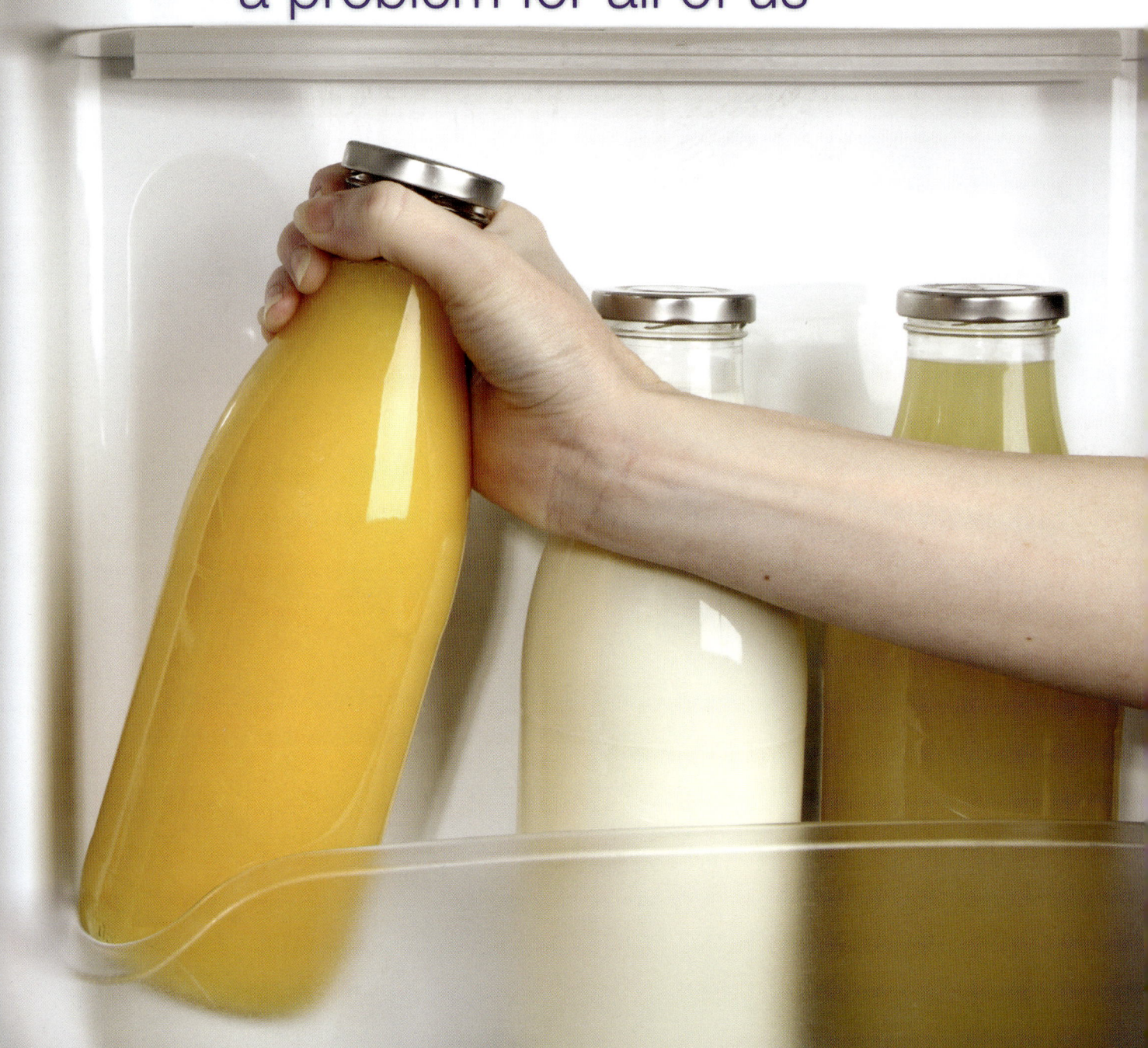

Chapter 3: Nutritional Considerations

Before you get started on the Food Guide, here is a bit of information about nutritional issues I have taken into account in devising the guide, and some ideas for other strategies that can help you.

Eating little and often

Most dieters report that the more diets they have been on, the harder it is to lose weight. When you think about it from an evolutionary point of view, it makes sense. Think of it this way: the more famines we live through, the more important it is for survival that our bodies become energy efficient – which means holding onto body fat as long as possible. This is a good reason to avoid cutting your Calorie intake too low without some expert advice.

It also makes sense to make the best use of your metabolism by dividing your food evenly over the day. I have devised this program using three meals and three snacks; this prevents you from becoming excessively hungry, which can result in poor food decisions. The three meals and three snacks approach also affects blood glucose and cholesterol levels positively. For those who can't manage to get those snacks in during the day, add the snacks evenly to the meals – don't keep all the extra Calories until the evening.

A balanced diet

Minimum daily nutritional requirements can be covered by:

- 2 pieces of fruit
- 4 slices of bread or ½ cup serves of cereal, rice, pasta or starchy vegetables
- 4 oz / 120 g meat or vegetarian protein
- 3 dairy serves
- 3 tsp oil or spread
- 2 ½ cups of 'free' vegetables.

Developing a meal plan structure can help to ensure you cover your needs. Here is one way that you can meet all your needs on even the lowest Calorie intake:

- Breakfast: cereal, milk and fruit
- AM snack: fruit
- Lunch: sandwich with meat and salad
- PM snack: dairy-based snack
- Dinner: meat, vegetables and either starchy vegetables, rice or pasta
- Supper snack: dairy-based snack.

When Calorie intake increases to maintenance level it becomes easier to reach this optimum nutritional intake while leaving space for some less healthy options.

Use the blank meal plan in Appendix 4 (see right) to plan your own routine.

PORTION PERFECTION | 27

Along with healthy eating, regular physical activity can help to manage and maintain a healthy weight.

These are the same principles applied in this book, so you can be confident that following the *Portion Perfection - A visual weight control plan* guide will contribute to positive outcomes in diabetes prevention and control. For further assistance, or if you are taking insulin or medication for either Type 2 or Type 1 diabetes, consult your Accredited Practising Dietitian.

What other strategies could you employ?

To help achieve your goal of weight loss, maintaining your weight or just eating healthily, in addition to following the guides shown in this book, you could:

1. Use the Portion Perfection Plate and Bowl routinely.

2. CalorieKing has created a simple and effective app for use in the US - see the app store for Control My Weight while My Fitness Pal is great for the UK food database.

3. Keep a food diary — we recommend Allan Borushek's *The CalorieKing Food & Exercise Journal*, available from **www.portiondiet.com**.

4. Break leftovers down into appropriate portions.

5. Buy smaller packages, focusing on those that contain a single serve per pack, or break down bulk packages as soon as you get them home into portioned amounts.

6. Develop a healthy attitude toward portion control. Try reading Dr Rick Kausman's book *If Not Dieting Then What?* Change needs to be permanent. Dr George Blair West's book, *Weight Loss for Food Lovers: Understanding our minds and why we sabotage our weight loss*, presents another useful approach. See our book list at **www.portiondiet.com** for more recommended books on nutrition and eating.

7. Work exercise into your routine so that it isn't a chore. We recommend 30 minutes of aerobic activity daily for weight loss, although more may be required to sustain a significant weight loss. We also recommend muscle-toning exercise to maintain strength and metabolic rate. For more information on setting up a healthy exercise program consult an exercise physiologist or speak to your doctor.

8. Use our great *4 Week Weight Loss Menu Plan* to plan your meals, or use any healthy cookbook along with the guides in this book to go it alone.

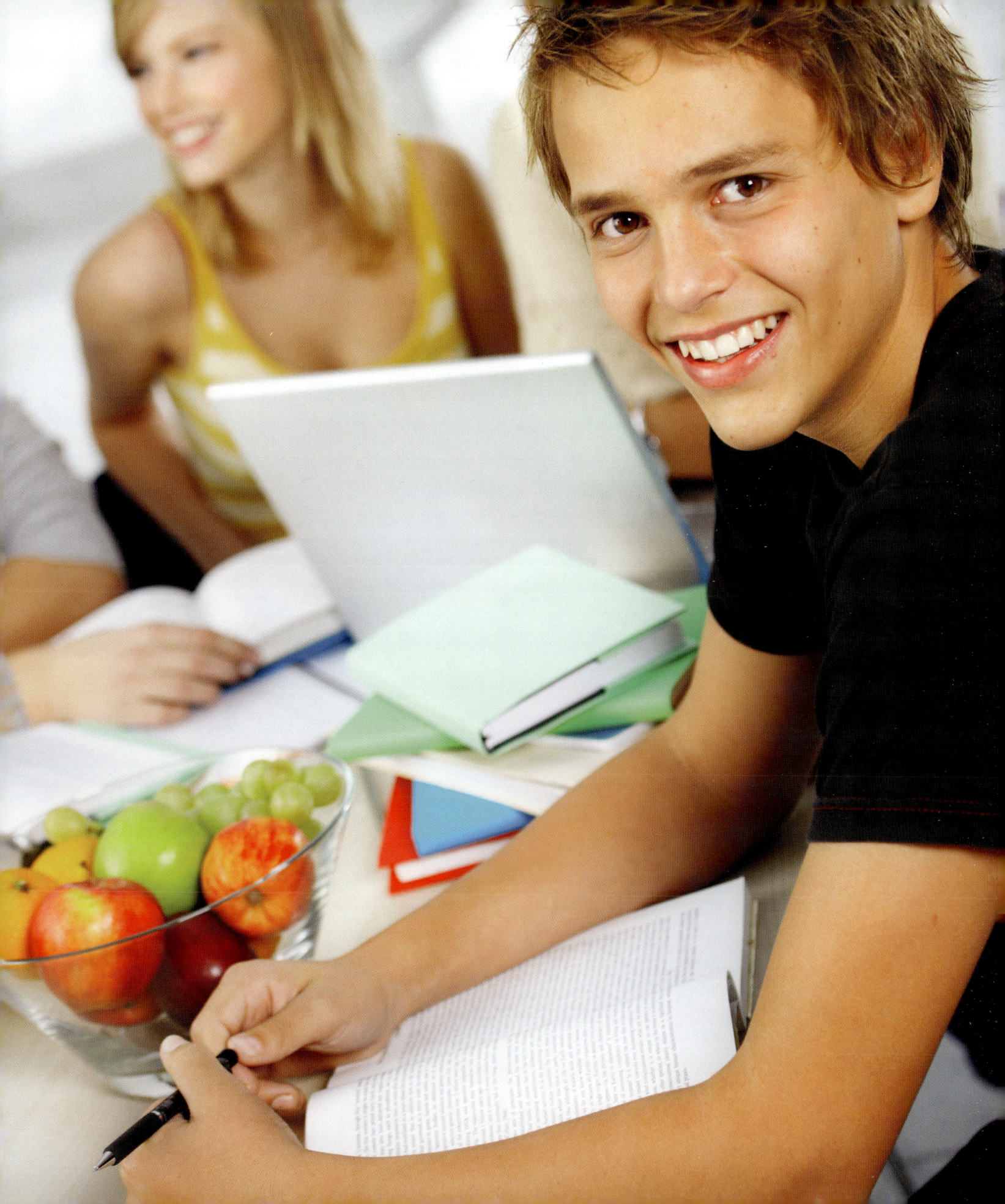

Chapter 4: Portion Perfection in Practice

In the following section, pictures are used to show you what to eat for each meal, based on recommended Calorie intake. For snacks, we recommend purchasing foods in discrete portions as close as possible to those represented in our snack pages.

What weight is right for me?

A simple way to assess your ideal weight is by using the Body Mass Index (BMI). This is a general measure of body fat, and provides a good general guide to whether you are underweight, average, or overweight. Higher BMIs result in higher risk for diabetes, heart disease and joint problems.

Calculate your BMI using one of the following equations:

Your weight (pounds) $\div$ your height (inches)^2 and multiply this answer by 703 = your BMI (kg/m^2)
OR *Your weight (kg) $\div$ your height (m)^2 = your BMI*

BMI 18.5–25 = Healthy weight
BMI 25–30 = Moderate health risk
BMI 30+ = High to very high health risk

Note: The BMI is useful as a general guide, however it does not take an individual's muscle mass into consideration. For a true assessment of your ideal weight, consult a qualified dietitian.

> **Recognizing a Qualified Dietitian**
>
> In the USA, look for a Registered Dietitian, in the UK, dietitians must be registered with the Health Care Professions Council and in Australia dietitians are Accredited. Some Australian dietitians, including the author, have been granted Advanced status for their professional achievements.

How much do I need?

The daily Calorie guide that this book is based on is as follows:

	Women and inactive teens	Men and active teens
To lose weight	1300 Cals / 5460 kJ ✓	1600 Cals / 6720 kJ ✓
To maintain weight	1800 Cals / 7560 kJ ✓	2200 Cals / 9240 kJ ✓

Note the colour that applies to your Calorie level and follow the corresponding coloured ticks throughout the food guide.

Children

Please note that weight loss in children can result in slowed growth. The best approach is to feed your child the correct amount and allow them to grow into their weight.

A dietitian can assist in situations where true loss of weight is required and we recommend you consult a qualified dietitian in your area. To find one in the US go to www.eatright.org and click on Find a Registered Dietitian. In the UK go to www.freelancedietitians.org and in Australia go to www.daa.asn.au and click on Find an APD or talk to your doctor.

For weight maintenance, an average Calorie requirement for 5–8 year olds is 1300 Cals / 5460 kJ. For 9-12 year olds it is 1600 Cals / 6720 kJ.

If weight loss results even when a child is adhering to recommended Calorie intake for weight maintenance, we recommend increasing the Calorie intake or consulting an APD.

Dividing it all up

It's not just about the total Calorie intake per day, it's also about the spacing of your meals. Ideally you should leave approximately two-and-a-half hours between a meal and a snack.

Your daily requirements	Breakfast Cals / kJ	Morning snack Cals / kJ	Lunch Cals / kJ	Afternoon snack Cals / kJ	Dinner Cals / kJ	Supper snack Cals / kJ
1300 Cals / 5460 kJ	300 / 1260	100 / 420	350 / 1470	100 / 420	350 / 1470	100 / 420
1600 Cals / 6720 kJ	400 / 1680	100 / 420	450 / 1890	100 / 420	450 / 1890	100 / 420
1800 Cals / 7560 kJ	400 / 1680	200 / 840	450 / 1890	200 / 840	450 / 1890	100 / 420
2200 Cals / 9240 kJ	500 / 2100	200 / 840	550 / 2310	200 / 840	550 / 2310	200 / 840
Custom____Cals						

Everyone is a little different when it comes to metabolism, so if you find that you are not achieving what you set out to do, step up or down a level. Alternatively, you can consult a qualified dietitian who will completely personalise the book for you by entering individualised recommendations in the preceding table.

For those who don't lose weight on 1300 Cals / 5460 kJ due to a slow metabolism, please either see a qualified dietitian to ensure your diet is balanced, or use a meal replacement to temporarily lower your intake of Calories.

Please note that lowering Calories below 1100 Cals / 4620 kJ per day may prove to be detrimental to your long-term ability to manage weight.

The inexact science of weight loss

To result in weight loss we need to consume fewer Calories than we are burning off. We tend not to do exactly the same amount of activity every day, but as long as our intake is less than our expenditure, then weight loss should result. This allows us to make the generalisations that most people will lose weight on the plan in this book. Some will lose weight faster than others, some slower, depending on exercise.

Maintaining weight is perhaps a bit more exact – to maintain, we need roughly equal energy intake and output. The plan in this book is a pretty good guide, but you may find you need to swap some snacks back to 100 Cals / 420 kJ, or you may need to increase portion sizes to meet your individual needs. For example when Brian (see the case study on page 24) reached his goal weight he moved to an intake of 2200 Calories / 9240 kJ, however he continued to lose weight slowly. We then added another 'Add Ons' serve (see Appendix 2) to his lunch and dinner, which resulted in weight maintenance.

If you have specific needs or metabolic problems, we encourage you to consult a qualified dietitian who will be able to review your profile and personalise your plan.

How to read food labels

Nutrition information labeling requirements vary between countries but the things that mislead us are universal. It is difficult to suggest the right nutritional content per serve because each company determines their own serving size and often it doesn't relate to a size that we would perceive to be one serve.

Where a "per 100g" set of data is provided, use this to compare between products to choose the better one.

Use the per serve figures to decide whether the number of Calories in the serve are right for your needs and check whether their statement of a serve size is realistic.

The product labels shown on the next page are in Australian, US and UK formats for the same product. Note for each of them that the container holds 5 serves.

Nutrition Information:		
Servings Per Package: 5		
Serving Size (40g)		
	Avg. Quantity per serving	Avg. Quantity per 100g
Energy	470kJ	1175kJ
Protein	1.4g	3.5g
Fat Total	8.5g	21.2g
– Saturated Fat	5.5g	13.7g
Carbohydrate	7.8g	19.5g
– Sugars	7.6g	19.0g
Sodium	19mg	48mg

Australian label

Nutrition Facts	
Serving Size 1 Tbsp (40g)	
Servings Per Container 5	
Amount Per Serving	
Calories 110	Calories from Fat 77
	% Daily Value
Total Fat 8.5g	13%
Saturated Fat 5.5g	27%
Cholesterol 30mg	10%
Sodium 19mg	1%
Total Carbohydrate 7.8g	3%
Dietary Fiber 0g	0%
Sugars 7.6g	
Protein 1.4g	
Vitamin A	4%
Vitamin C	0%
Calcium	15%
Iron	2%

US label

per 40g dessert:

| 5 SERVINGS | ENERGY 460kJ 110kcal 6% | FAT 8.5g MED 13% | SATURATES 5.5g HIGH 27% | SUGARS 7.6g HIGH 9% | SALT 0.01g LOW 1% |

% of an adult's reference intake.
Typical values per 100g: Energy 1175kJ/280kcal

UK label

Decide whether this food is a meal or a snack and check your Calorie target and remember the goal of 200–250 Cals / 840-1050 kJ for meals and 100 Cals / 420 kJ for snacks.

What else is on the label?

You'll also find on the label information about:

- **Protein**: Protein helps you feel more satisfied and keeps your blood sugar levels steady. Your daily requirement is likely to be 50–80 g. This figure will give you a feel for whether the product is a good source of protein or not. The pictured product is fairly low in protein, at 1.4 g per serve.

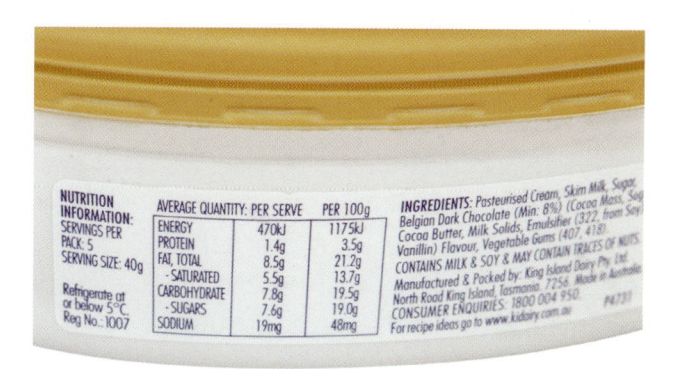

PORTION PERFECTION | 35

- **Fat**: This is often broken down into total fat and saturated fat, while some products may also list unsaturated fats and omega 3 fatty acids. In general you want no more than one-third of the fat in the food to be saturated. A low-fat food contains less than 3 g fat per 100 g of food. A low-fat meal is generally made up of foods that total not more than 10 g of fat and a suitable snack would have no more than 5 g of fat. The pictured product is a little high in fat for an everyday snack, and the fat is primarily saturated. If consumed in the ideal Calorie amount, then this could be an occasional snack (see page 29 for more details on occasional snacks and everyday foods).

- **Carbohydrate**: This is broken down into total carbohydrate and sugars. One trick is that the 'sugars' figure includes naturally occurring sugars in any fruit in the product as well as any milk ingredient. You will need to look at the ingredient list to get a feel for where the sugar is coming from. In general look for less than 5 g of added sugar for a snack or less than 10 g for a meal. Higher sugar intakes can be acceptable if there is more than 2 g of fibre in the snack or if it is based on fruit. The carbohydrate reading is not a good indicator of the glycemic index of a food.

  The pictured product contains 7.8 g of carbohydrate, of which 7.6 g is sugar. This is a milk-based product so we know some of that sugar is actually the lactose in the milk. If you refer back to the GI chart on page 28, you will see that most dairy products are low GI even when they have added sugar. The sugar is therefore absorbed fairly slowly, making this a 'safer' source of sugar.

- **Fibre**: High fibre foods generally have higher nutritional value and lower GI. Look for products with more than 3 g of fibre per 100 g, or more than 8 g per 100 g for breakfast cereals. The pictured product does not contain a fibre listing for the Australian and UK labels and shows 0 g on the US product label. Being a milk product, this food would not be expected to contain significant fibre.

- **Sodium**: This is important for those on a sodium-restricted diet. Foods are considered to be low salt if they contain less than 120 mg sodium per 100 g of food. Moderate salt foods usually contain less than 450 mg sodium per 100 g of product. The pictured product would qualify as a low salt food.

There may be other nutritional components shown on the labels that you read; however, the ones listed in this section are the important ones for our purpose.

The ingredients list for this product includes Pasteurised Cream, Fat Free Milk, Belgian Dark Chocolate, Cocoa Butter, Milk Solids, Emulsifiers, Flavour and Vegetable Gums. Cream being the first ingredient on the list explains this product's high saturated fat content. The chemical content is quite low and most of the additives listed (vegetable gums and emulsifiers) are not commonly associated with any adverse reactions.

This product could be classified as an occasional food and a 100 Calorie / 420 kJ snack would be approximately one spoonful.

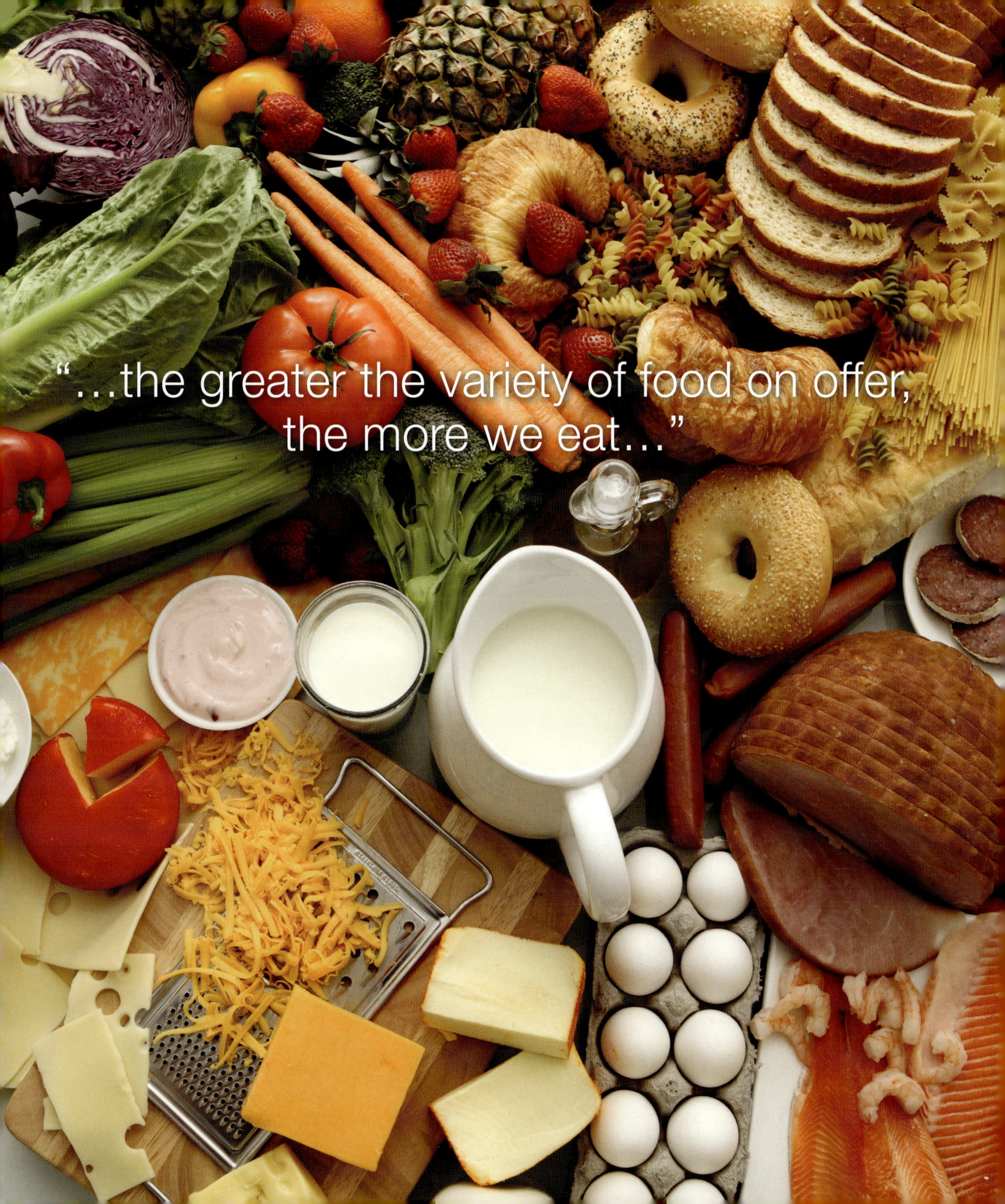

"...the greater the variety of food on offer, the more we eat..."

Chapter 5: Food guide basics

Welcome to the food guide. This section is divided into meals, starting with breakfast, and moving on through snacks, which include a morning, afternoon and supper snack, then onto lunch and dinner.

To get started:

1. Identify which Calorie intake is right for you using the table below. The colour codings in the table are used throughout, so familiarise yourself with your colour.

	Women and inactive teens	Men and active teens
To lose weight	1300 Cals / 5460 kJ ✓	1600 Cals / 6720 kJ ✓
To maintain weight	1800 Cals / 7560 kJ ✓	2200 Cals / 9240 kJ ✓

2. Move to the appropriate section of the Food Guide for the meal of choice, for example, breakfast on page 41.

3. Select a menu option (note the recommended limits on occasional choices on page 29), and turn to that page.

4. Note the appropriate portion serve for your recommended Calorie intake and prepare your meal accordingly.

> Everyday choices have a green border on the page and occasional choices have a purple border.

Note the hints and tips for recipe selection or use the *4 Week Weight Loss Menu Plan*.

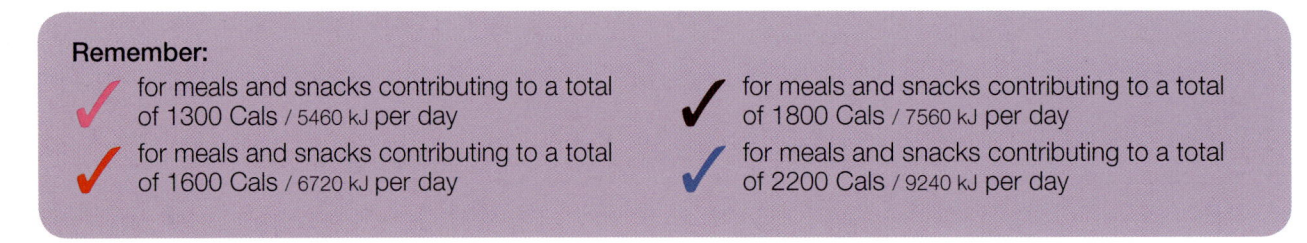

> **Remember:**
> ✓ for meals and snacks contributing to a total of 1300 Cals / 5460 kJ per day
> ✓ for meals and snacks contributing to a total of 1600 Cals / 6720 kJ per day
> ✓ for meals and snacks contributing to a total of 1800 Cals / 7560 kJ per day
> ✓ for meals and snacks contributing to a total of 2200 Cals / 9240 kJ per day

Now you're ready to perfect your portions! Enjoy!

"Enjoy a cool glass of water anytime."

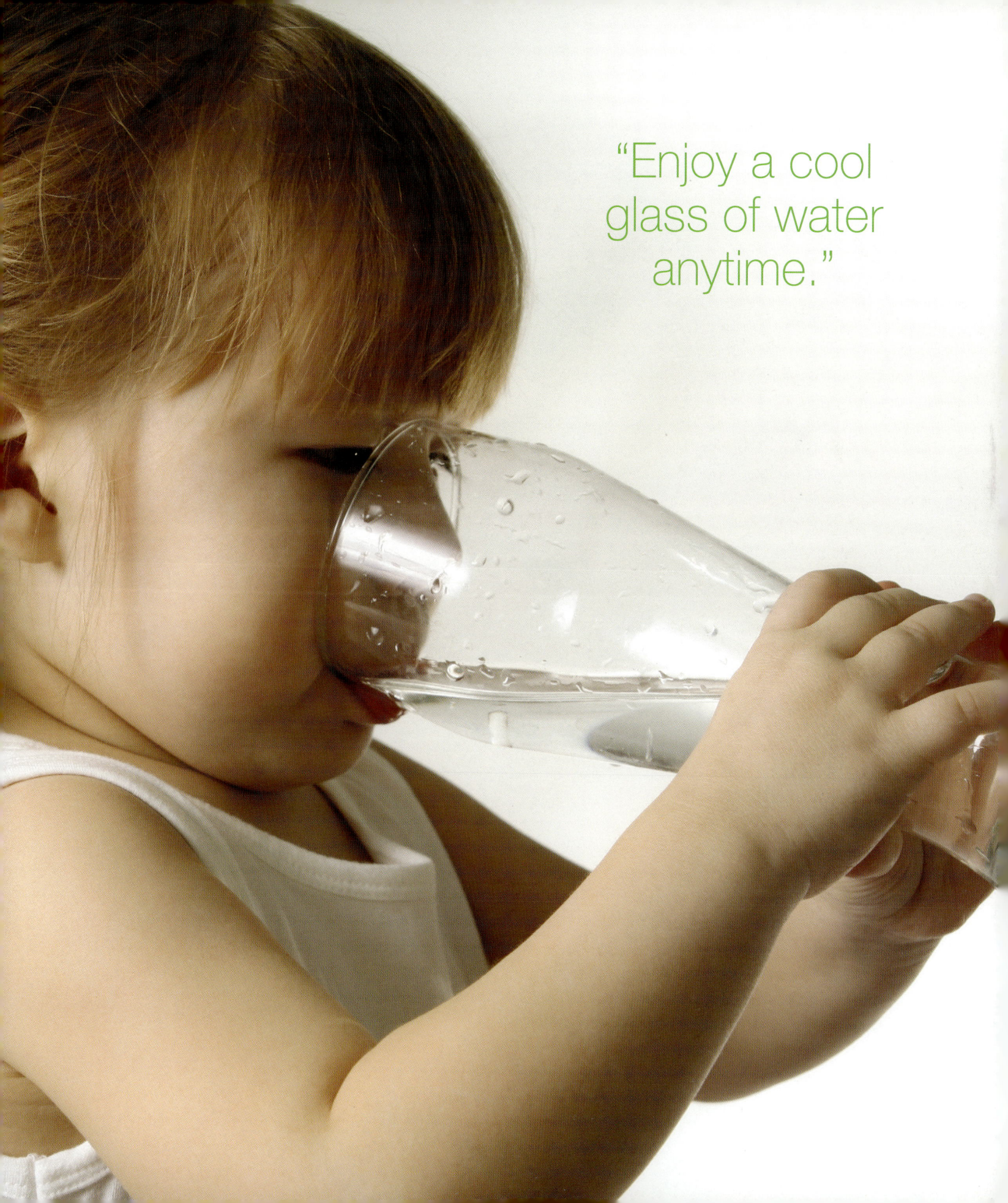

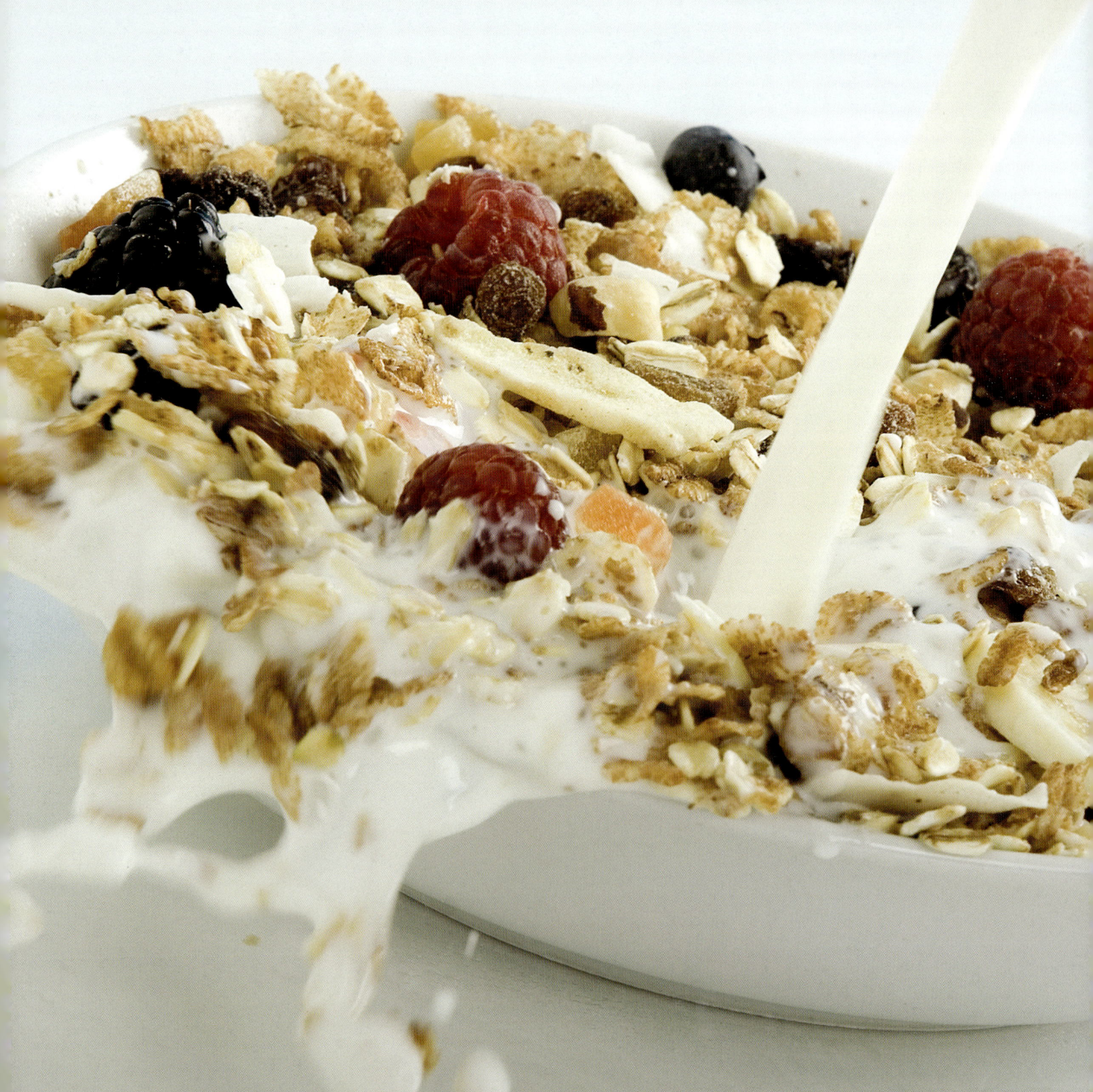

"...the larger the bowl the more we eat..."

CHAPTER 6

breakfast

This is the most socially acceptable time of day to eat fibre, so don't miss the boat. The highest fibre choice is a high-fibre cereal or baked beans on toast. Breakfast kick-starts the metabolism, and there is clear evidence that concentration levels are improved in the mornings following breakfast. We also know that those who skip breakfast end up eating more Calories over the course of the day than those who eat first thing in the morning.

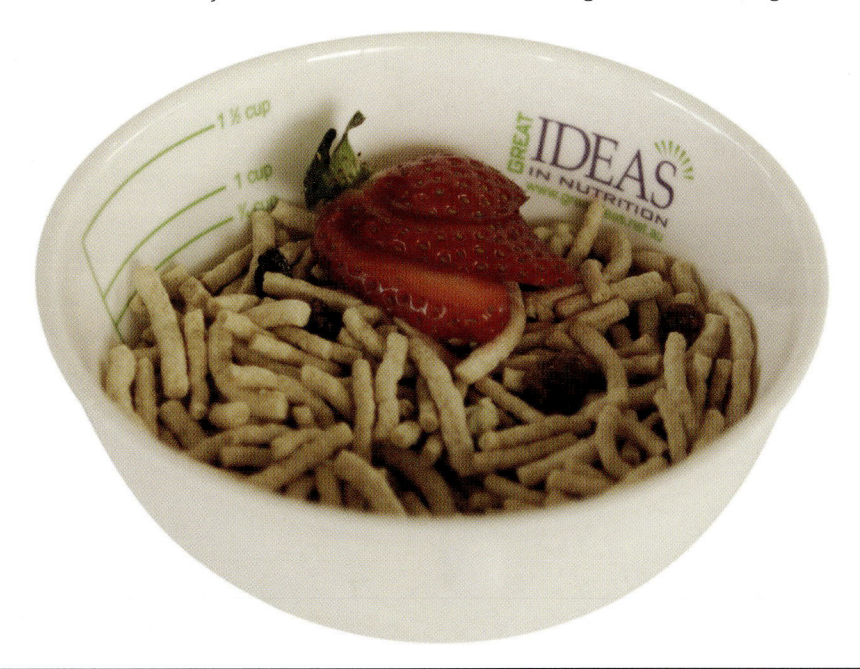

everyday menu

Toast & topping 42
Milk, fruit & cereal 44
Yoghurt & fruit... 48
Smoothie.. 50
Fruit salad.. 51
Omelette 52

occasional menu

Bacon & eggs... 54
Pancakes 55
Crumpets 56
Bagels... 57
Croissant... 58
Fast food... 59
Waffles 60
Donut 61

Add your own favourites by calculating the appropriate serve from Allan Borushek's *The CalorieKing Calorie Fat and Carbohydrate Counter* **or apps CalorieKing or My Fitness Pal.**

BREAKFAST | 41

everyday breakfast

toast & toppings

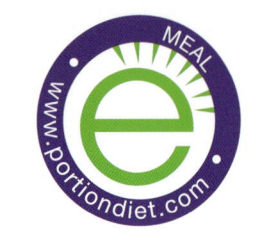

Toast can be a great way to start the day, but is it Calorie-wise to have juice and a Macchiato with it? Consider the components of a toast-based breakfast to be the bread, the toppings and drinks that accompany the toast (Add Ons), and other choices that won't significantly add to the Calories but enhance the meal. Refer to the table below to determine the right amount for you. For example, a 300 Calorie / 1260 kJ breakfast could consist of 2 slices of wholegrain toast, ½ cup cottage cheese and sliced tomato.

Meal components

Cals / kJ	Breads (100 Cals / 420 kJ)	Add Ons (100 Cals / 420 kJ)	Free Foods (<20 Cals / 85 kJ)
300 / 1260 ✓	2	1	1
400 / 1680 ✓✓	2	2	2
500 / 2100 ✓	3	2	2

Toast (100 Cals / 420 kJ)

Lower GI

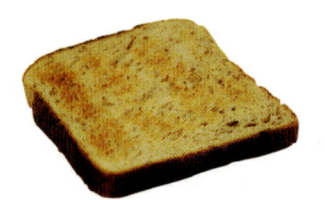

Wholegrain bread, 1 slice, 1 oz / 30 g

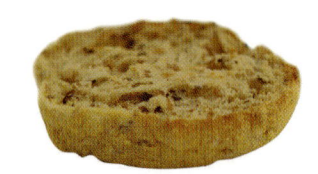

Wholegrain or fruit English muffin, ½

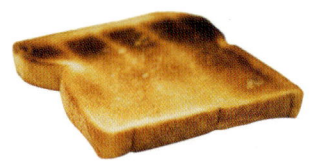

Low GI white bread, 1 slice, 1 oz / 30 g

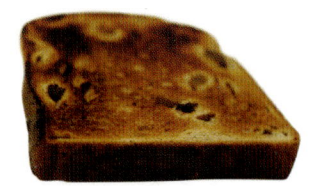

Raisin bread, 1 slice, 1 oz / 30 g

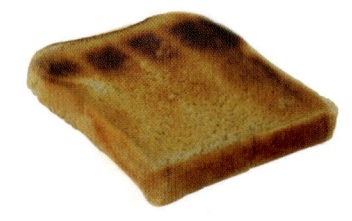

Stoneground wholemeal or sourdough rye, 1 slice, 1 oz / 30 g

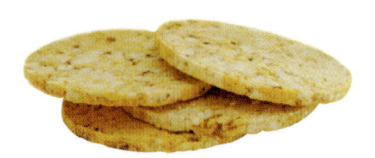

Grainy corn / rice cakes, 4

Higher GI

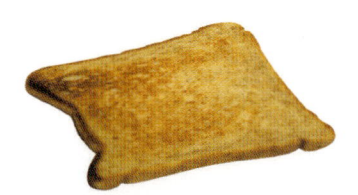

Whole wheat bread, 1 slice, 1 oz / 30 g

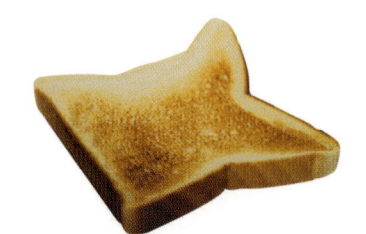

White bread, 1 slice, 1 oz / 30 g

TIP

Learn to count Calories by the 100s. 100 Cals / 420 kJ in each slice of bread, 100 Cals / 420 kJ in each 'Add On', 100 Cals / 420 kJ in each food in the 100 Cal snack lists.

everyday breakfast

toast & toppings continued

Add Ons (100 Cals / 420 kJ)

*For more 'Add Ons' serves refer to Appendix 2

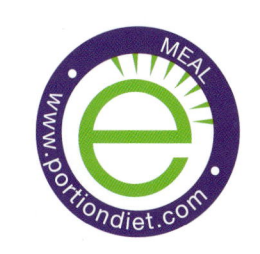

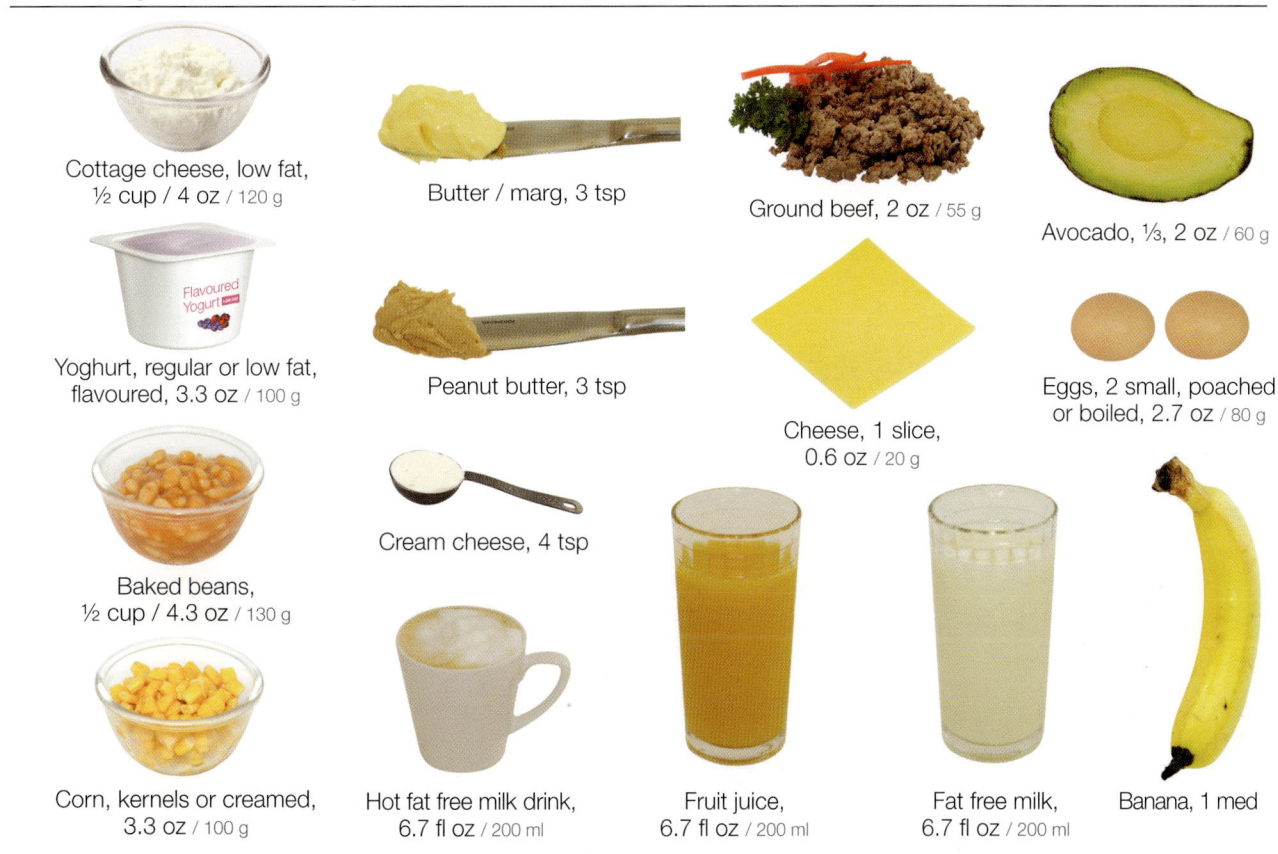

Cottage cheese, low fat, ½ cup / 4 oz / 120 g

Butter / marg, 3 tsp

Ground beef, 2 oz / 55 g

Avocado, ⅓, 2 oz / 60 g

Yoghurt, regular or low fat, flavoured, 3.3 oz / 100 g

Peanut butter, 3 tsp

Cheese, 1 slice, 0.6 oz / 20 g

Eggs, 2 small, poached or boiled, 2.7 oz / 80 g

Baked beans, ½ cup / 4.3 oz / 130 g

Cream cheese, 4 tsp

Corn, kernels or creamed, 3.3 oz / 100 g

Hot fat free milk drink, 6.7 fl oz / 200 ml

Fruit juice, 6.7 fl oz / 200 ml

Fat free milk, 6.7 fl oz / 200 ml

Banana, 1 med

Free foods (< 20 Cals / 85 kJ)

*For more 'free food' serves refer to Appendix 3

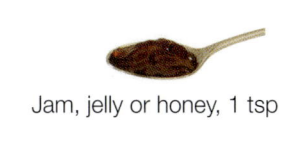

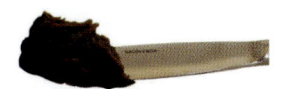

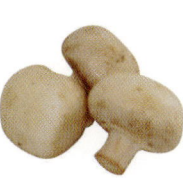

Jam, jelly or honey, 1 tsp

Mushrooms, 3 med, 2 oz / 60 g

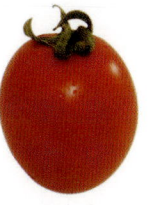

Tomato, 1 med, 3.3 oz / 100 g

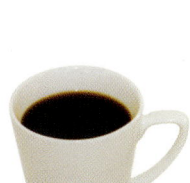

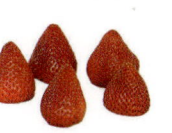

Strawberries, 5

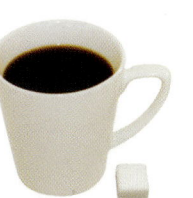

Enjoy anytime

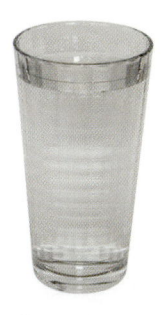

Yeast extract, 2 tsp

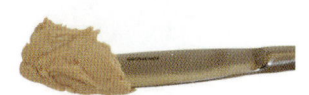

Deviled ham or meat spread, 2 tsp

Asparagus spears, 5

Tea/coffee, black/white with milk or 1 sugar

Glass of water

BREAKFAST | 43

everyday breakfast

milk, fruit & cereal

The following cereal estimates contain 150 Calories / 630 kJ per serve. Compare your cereal to the nutritional criteria below and then identify the picture that most closely resembles your cereal to determine the recommended volume.

Meal components

Cals / kJ	Milk (100 Cals / 420 kJ)	Fruit (50 Cals / 210 kJ)	Cereal (150 Cals / 630 kJ)	Free (optional) (<20 Cals / 85 kJ)
300 / 1260 ✓	1	1	1	1
400 / 1680 ✓✓	1	1.5	1.5	1
500 / 2100 ✓	1.5	1	2	1

Cereal Criteria

Because cereals have varying serving sizes listed on the pack, for the assessment of whether a cereal is healthy enough to consume every day I recommend the CalorieKing app in the US and Australia or My Fitness Pal in the UK. Choose your cereal, enter a serve size of 100 g and check the following criteria. Some countries may indicate the nutritional data for a 100 g serve on the label.

1. Less than 14 g / 100 g sugar If no or very little fruit content OR Less than 28 g / 100 g of sugar if it contains significant fruit*
2. More than 8 g / 100 g fibre
3. Less than 4 g / 100 g saturated fat

* Considered to be 25% or more fruit content. If you have diabetes, choose cereals that meet all 3 criteria; for general health ensure cereals meet at least 2 of the criteria listed.

Milk (100 Cals / 420 kJ)

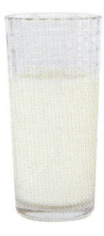

Whole milk, 5 fl oz / 150 ml

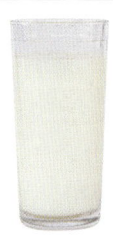

Reduced / low fat milk (1-2%), 6.7 fl oz / 200 ml

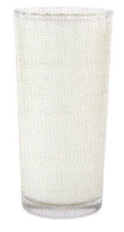

Skim milk, 7.3 fl oz / 220 ml

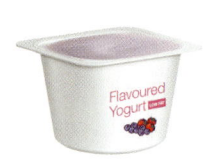

Yoghurt, regular or low fat, flavoured, 3.3 oz / 100 g

Fruit (50 Cals / 210 kJ)

*For more fruit serves refer to Appendix 1

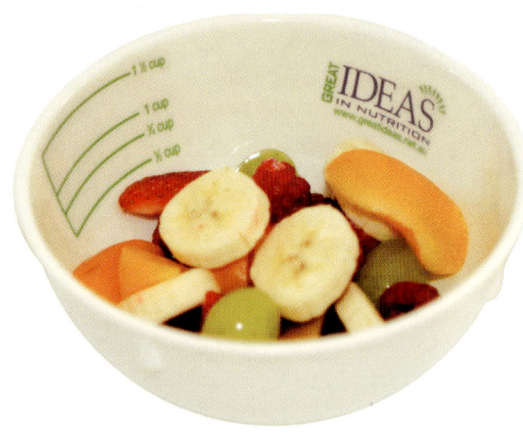

Fruit salad, ½ cup

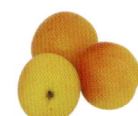

Apricots, 3

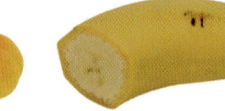

Banana, ½ med

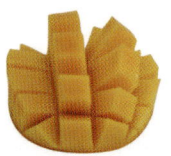

Mango, ½

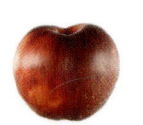

Nectarine, 1

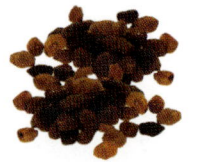

Raisins or Sultanas, 2 Tbsp, 0.6 oz / 20 g

TIP If constipation is a problem, consider replacing 1 fruit serve with an additional 2 serves of "free" fibre.

everyday breakfast

milk, fruit & cereal *continued*

After determining the suitability of your cereal choice, then use the guide below to recognise your cereal type.

1 serve = ¼ cup natural or toasted granola

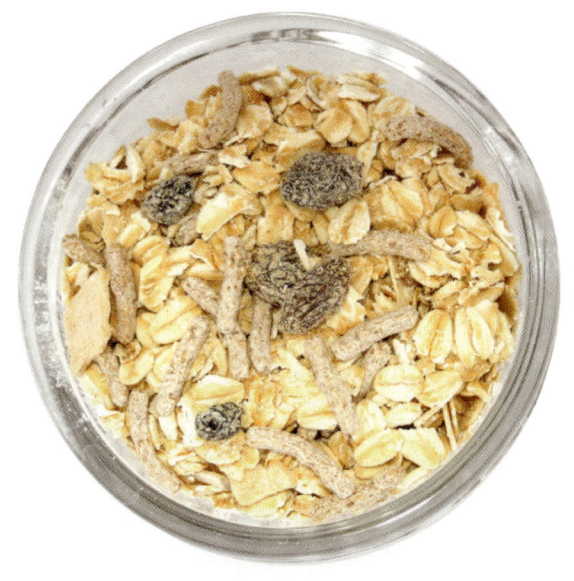

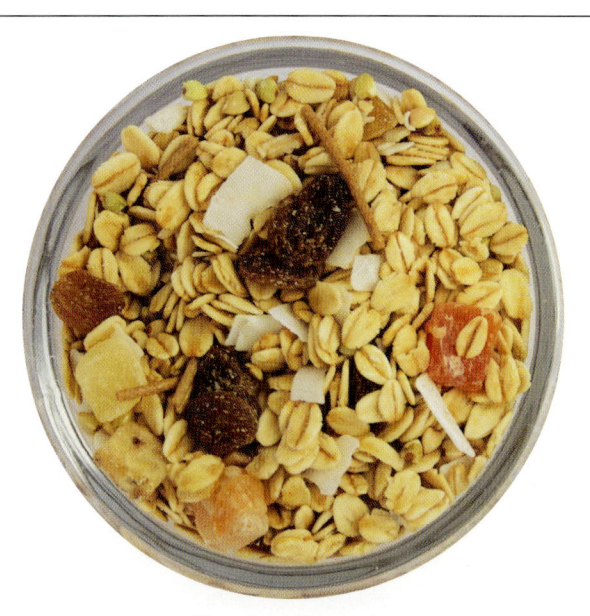

Natural Granola

Toasted Granola

1 serve = ½ cup (or 1.3 oz / 35 g packet) raw oats or clusters

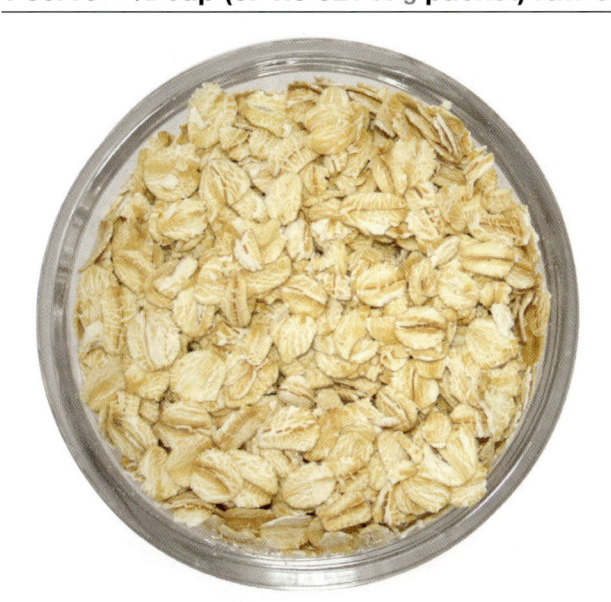

Raw Wholegrain or Steel Cut Oats

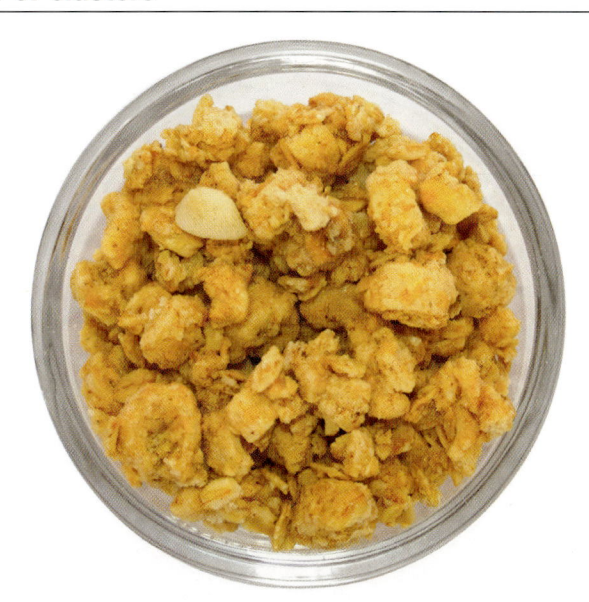

Cluster Cereal

Note: For sachet oats, look for whole or multigrain varieties.

Continued over ❱

BREAKFAST | 45

everyday breakfast

milk, fruit & cereal continued

1 serve = ¾ cup mixed cereals or bran

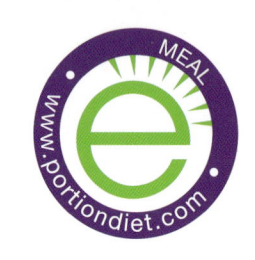

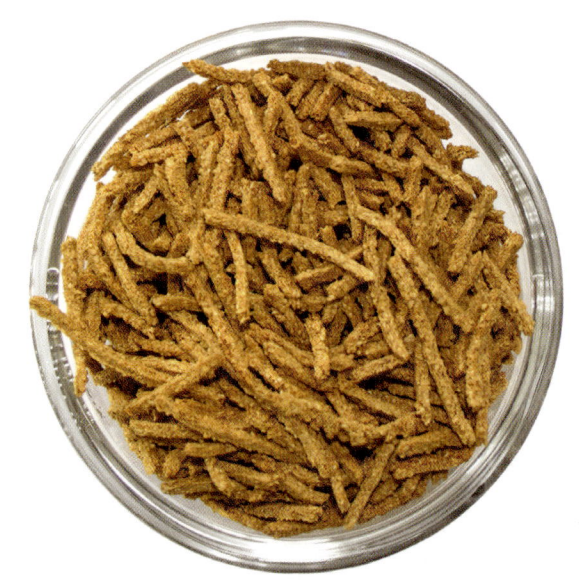

Processed Bran

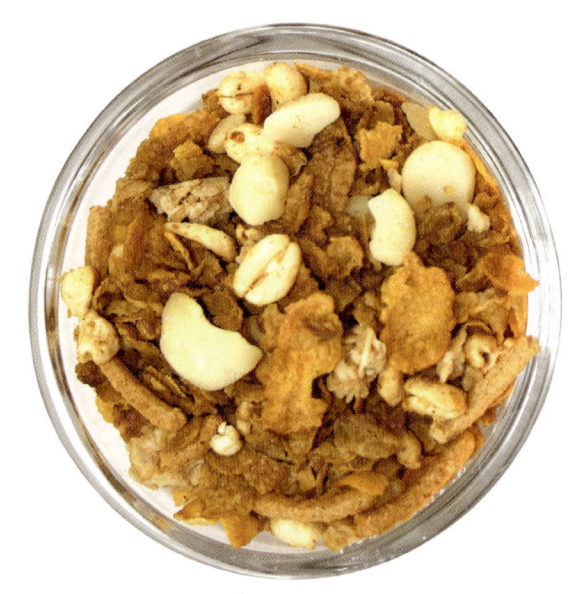

Fruit, Flakes and Nuts

1 serve = 1 cup light or flaky cereals

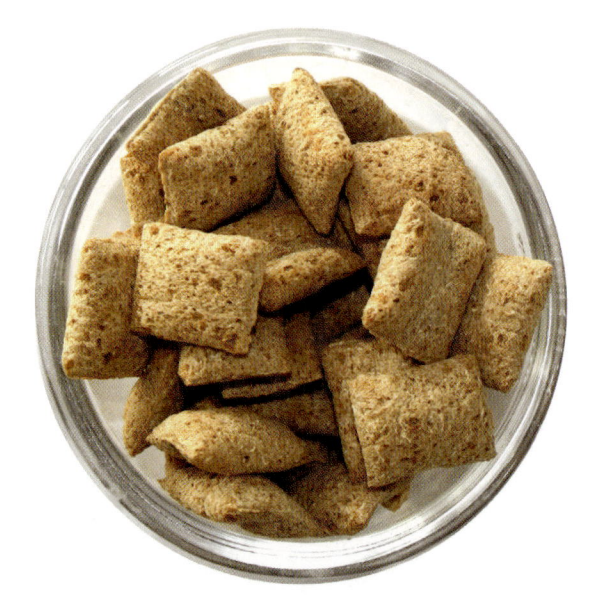

Light Cereals

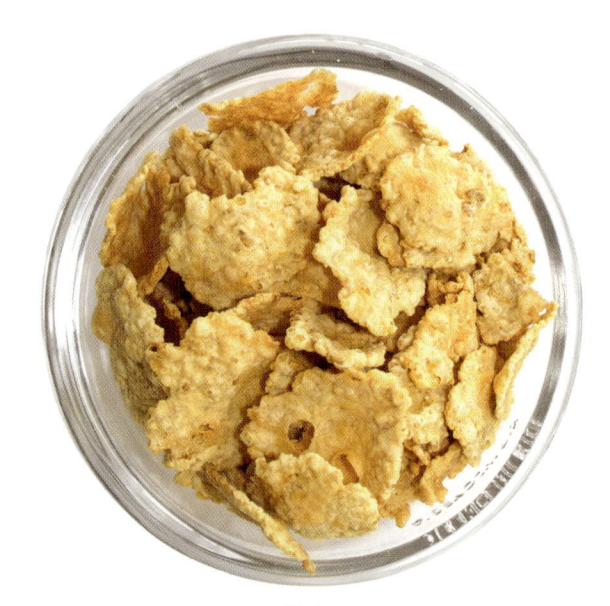

Flakes

everyday breakfast

milk, fruit & cereal *continued*

2 large or 16 mini breakfast biscuits

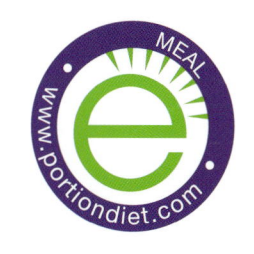

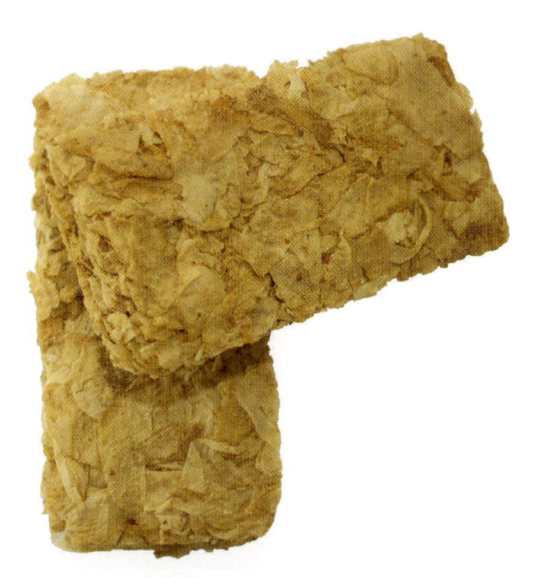

Breakfast Biscuits

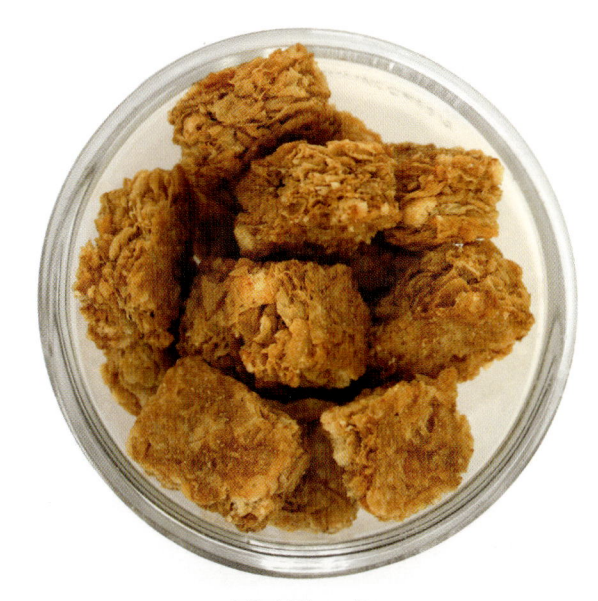

Mini Biscuits

Free Food – 1 Tbsp bran

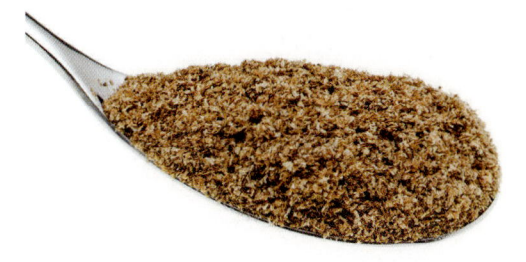

Bran – Oatbran, Psyllium, Wheatgerm, Unprocessed Bran

BREAKFAST | 47

everyday breakfast
yoghurt & fruit

Choose yoghurt and fruit serves according to the table below.

Meal components

Cals / kJ	Yoghurt (200 Cals / 840 kJ)	Fruit (50 Cals / 210 kJ)
300 / 1260 ✓	1	2
400 / 1680 ✓✓	1	4
500 / 2100 ✓	2	2

Yoghurt (200 Cals / 840 kJ)

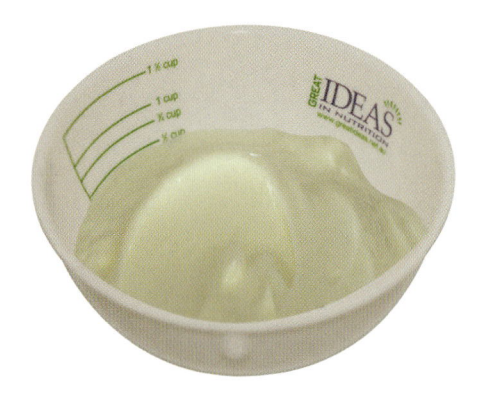

Greek style, ½ cup

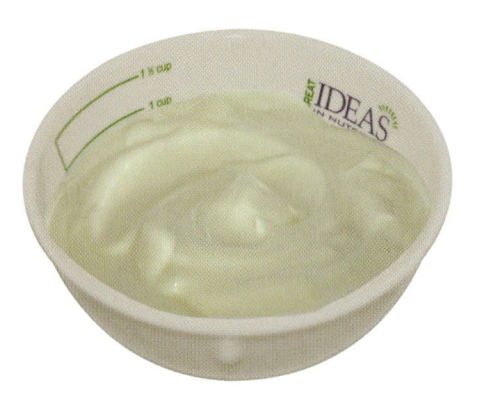

Greek style, no fat, 1 cup

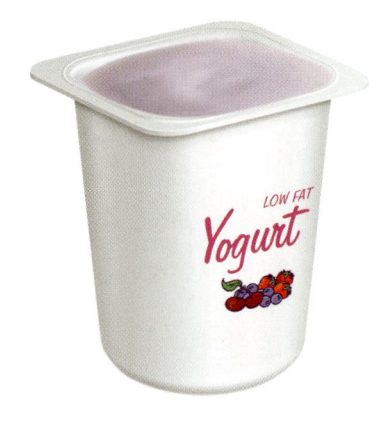

Low fat yoghurt, ⅔ cup, 6.7 oz / 200 g

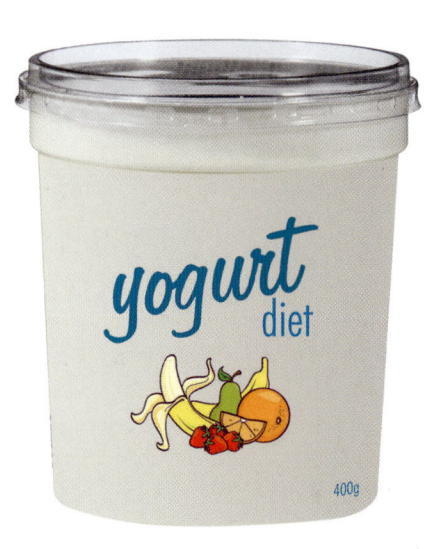

Low fat, artificially sweetened (diet) yoghurt, 1½ cups, 13.3 oz / 400 g

48 | BREAKFAST

everyday breakfast

yoghurt & fruit continued

Fruit (50 Cals / 210 kJ)

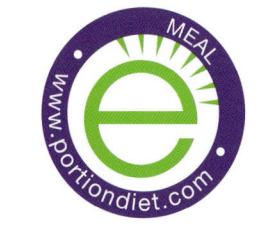

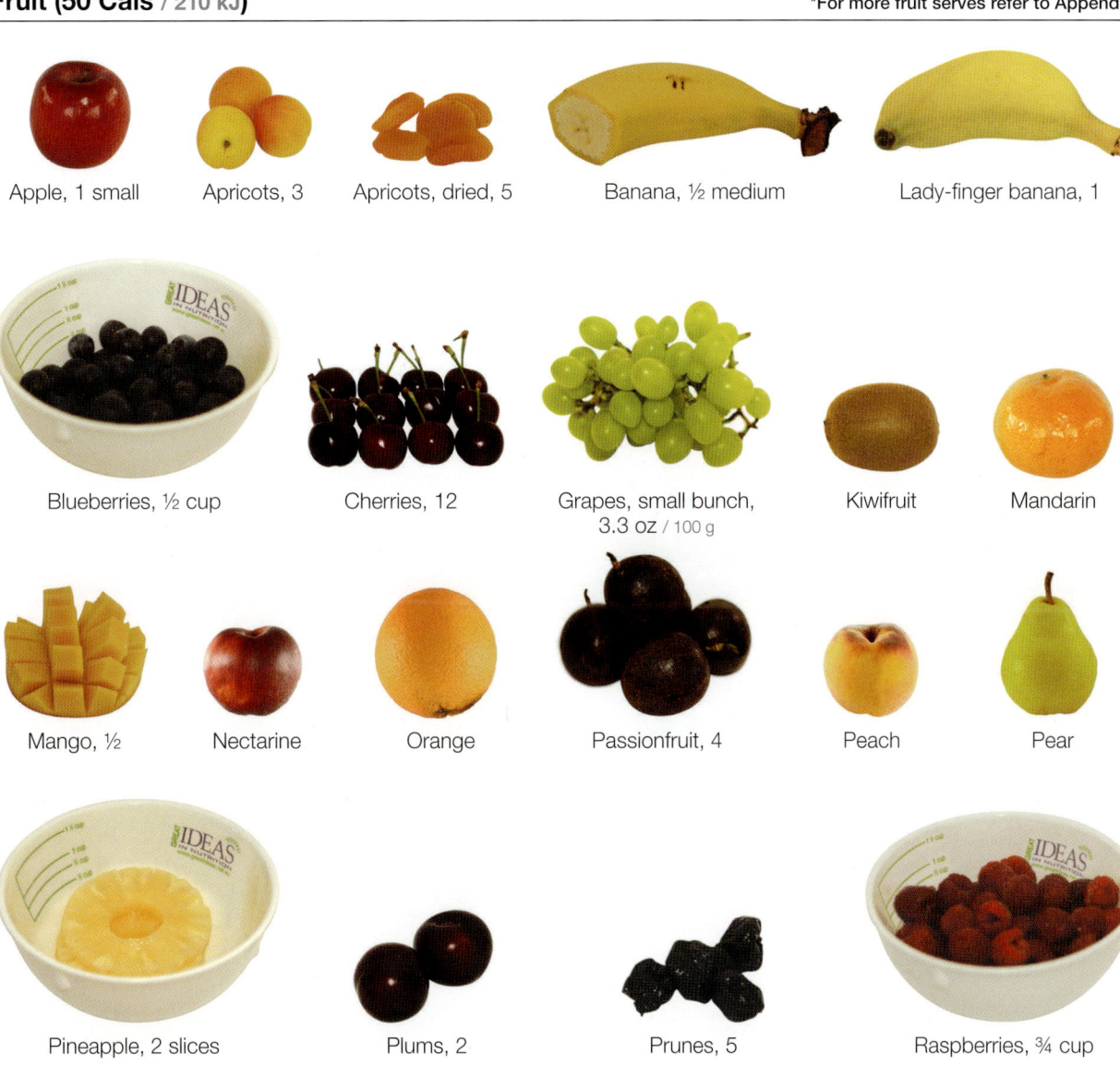

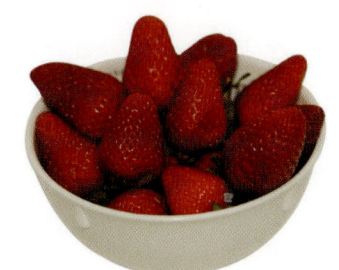

*For more fruit serves refer to Appendix 1

Apple, 1 small

Apricots, 3

Apricots, dried, 5

Banana, ½ medium

Lady-finger banana, 1

Blueberries, ½ cup

Cherries, 12

Grapes, small bunch, 3.3 oz / 100 g

Kiwifruit

Mandarin

Mango, ½

Nectarine

Orange

Passionfruit, 4

Peach

Pear

Pineapple, 2 slices

Plums, 2

Prunes, 5

Raspberries, ¾ cup

Strawberries, 1½ cups

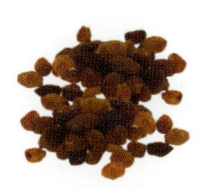

Raisins or Sultanas, 2 Tbsp, 0.6 oz / 20 g

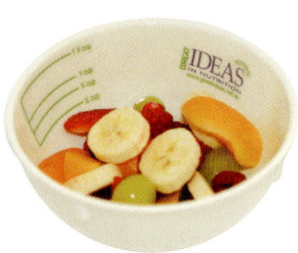

Fruit salad or canned fruit, ½ cup

BREAKFAST | 49

everyday breakfast
smoothie

A smoothie can be a great way to start the day. If buying one, ask for fat free milk and pay attention to the serving sizes below.

Meal components

Cals / kJ	Milk (100 Cals / 420 kJ)	Add Ons (100 Cals / 420 kJ)	Fruit (50 Cals / 210 kJ)
300 / 1260 ✓	1.5	1	1
400 / 1680 ✓✓	1.5	1.5	2
500 / 2100 ✓	2	2	2

Pictures shown here are based on low fat millk. See page 44 or Appendix 2 for serve sizes for fat free or whole milks. See page 49 or Appendix 1 for fruit serves.

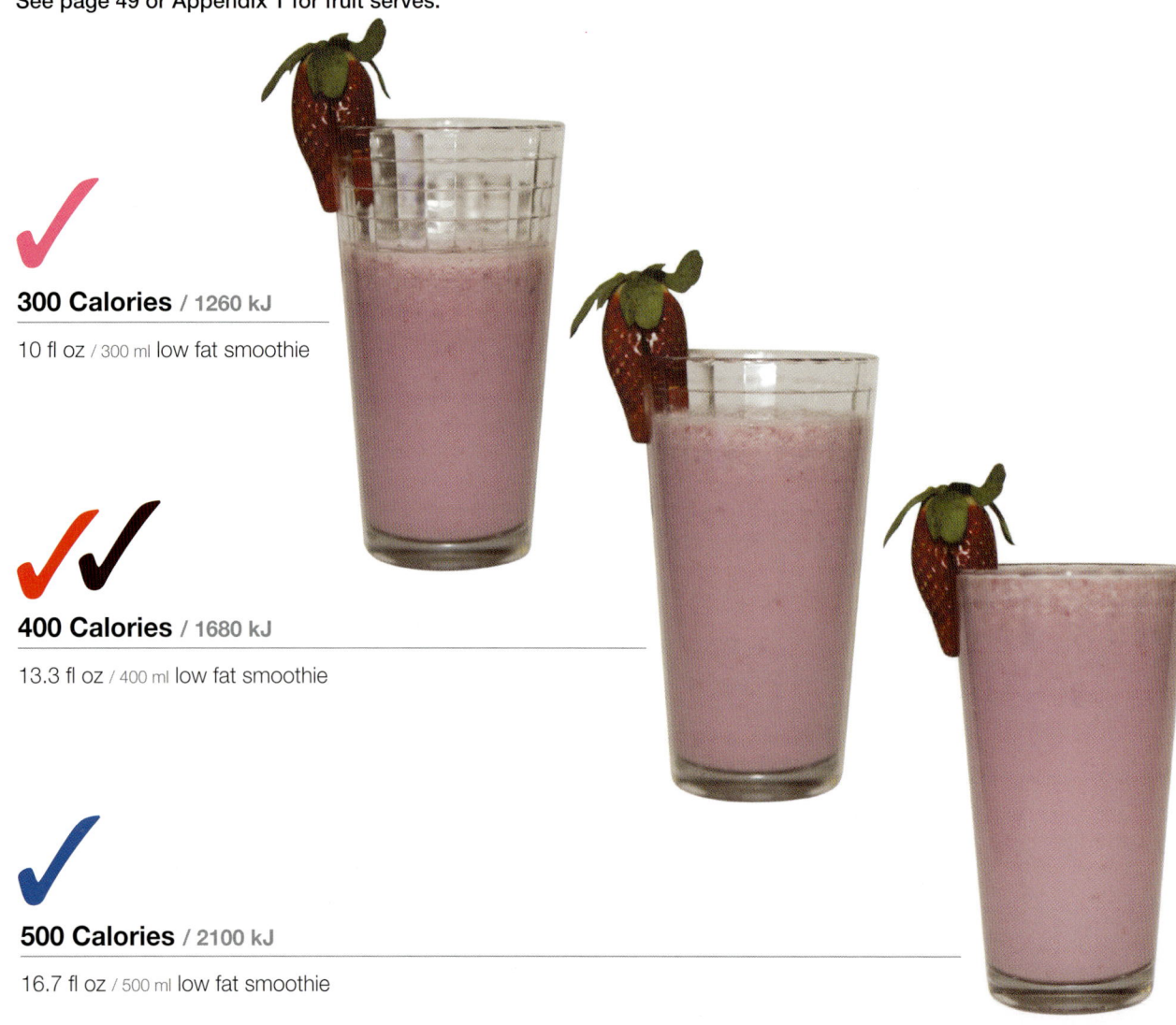

300 Calories / 1260 kJ

10 fl oz / 300 ml low fat smoothie

400 Calories / 1680 kJ

13.3 fl oz / 400 ml low fat smoothie

500 Calories / 2100 kJ

16.7 fl oz / 500 ml low fat smoothie

TIP If you like to add other ingredients to your smoothies such as oils or fibre, check the Calories and add to your Add Ons or Free Foods lists in the Appendix.

everyday breakfast
fruit salad

For fruit serves refer to page **49** or Appendix 1.

Meal components

Cals / kJ	Fruit (50 Cals / 210 kJ)
300 / 1260 ✓	6
400 / 1680 ✓✓	8
500 / 2100 ✓	10

✓ **300 Calories** / 1260 kJ
6 piece fruit salad

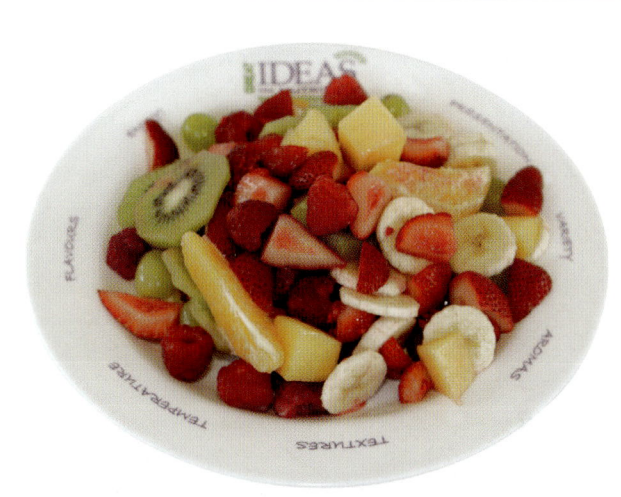

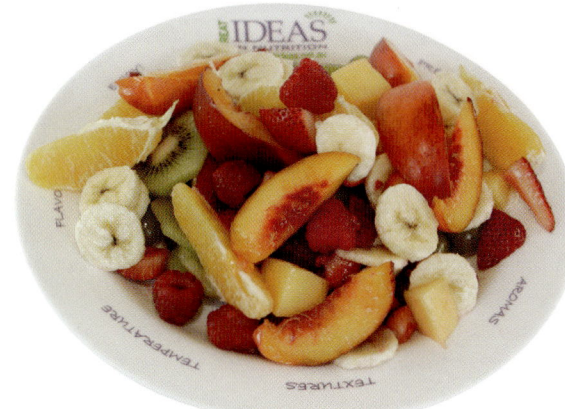

✓✓ **400 Calories** / 1680 kJ
8 piece fruit salad

✓ **500 Calories** / 2100 kJ
10 piece fruit salad

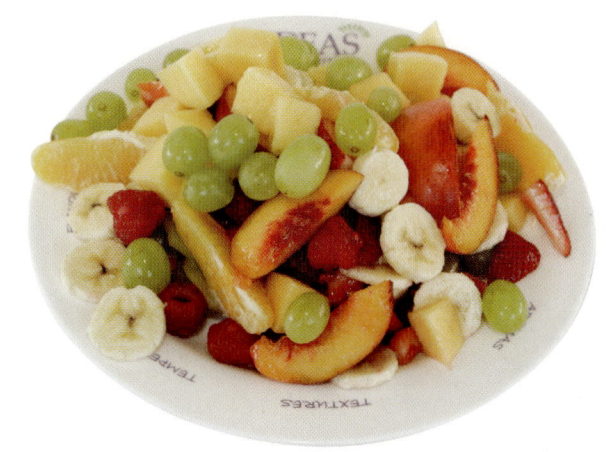

TIP A fruit-only breakfast can leave you unfulfilled; choosing an option that includes protein will be more satisfying.

BREAKFAST | 51

everyday breakfast
omelette

To make an omelette, whip eggs and about ¼ cup of milk per egg along with any fresh or dried herbs you like. Cook until dry on top, flip, and serve filled with the following ingredients.

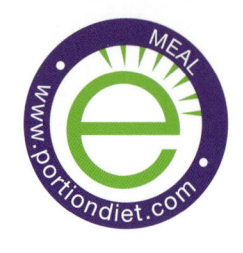

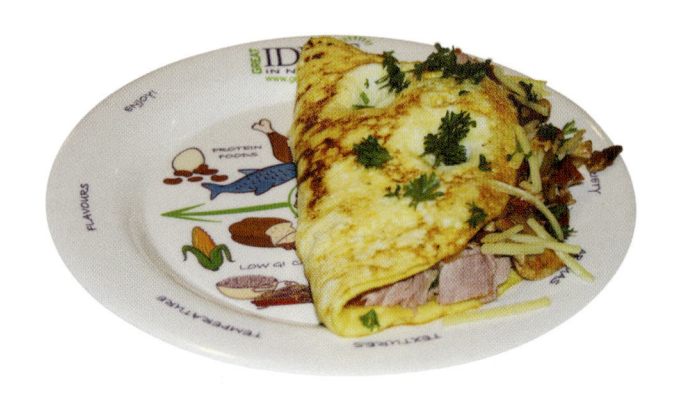

300 Calories / 1260 kJ

2 egg omelette (200 Cals / 840 kJ)
+ 0.3 oz / 10 g cheese (50 Cals / 210 kJ)
+ 1 tomato (30 Cals / 126 kJ)
+ 1 onion (12 Cals / 50 kJ)
+ 3 mushrooms (8 Cals / 32 kJ)

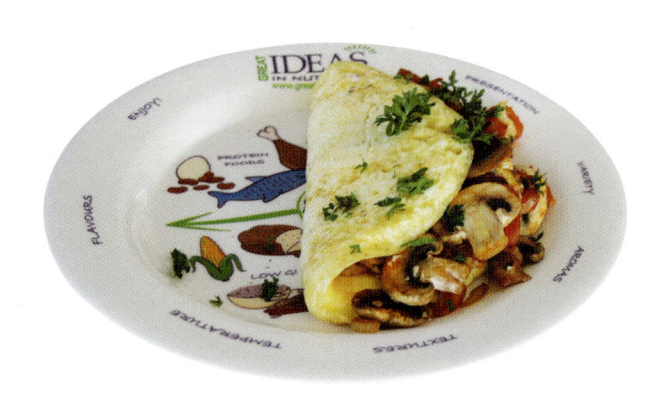

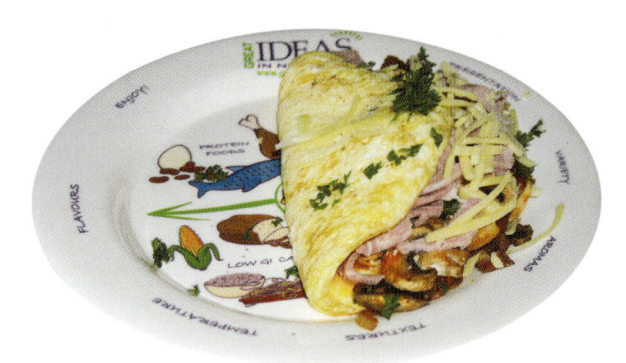

400 Calories / 1680 kJ

2 egg omelette (200 Cals / 840 kJ)
+ 0.7 oz / 20 g cheese (100 Cals / 420 kJ)
+ 1 tomato (30 Cals / 126 kJ)
+ 1 onion (12 Cals / 50 kJ)
+ 3 mushrooms (8 Cals / 32 kJ)
+ 1.3 oz / 40 g ham (50 Cals / 210 kJ)

500 Calories / 2100 kJ

3 egg omelette (300 Cals / 1260 kJ)
+ 0.7 oz / 20 g cheese (100 Cals / 420 kJ)
+ 1 tomato (30 Cals / 126 kJ)
+ 1 onion (12 Cals / 50 kJ)
+ 3 mushrooms (8 Cals / 32 kJ)
+ 1.3 oz / 40 g ham (50 Cals / 210 kJ)

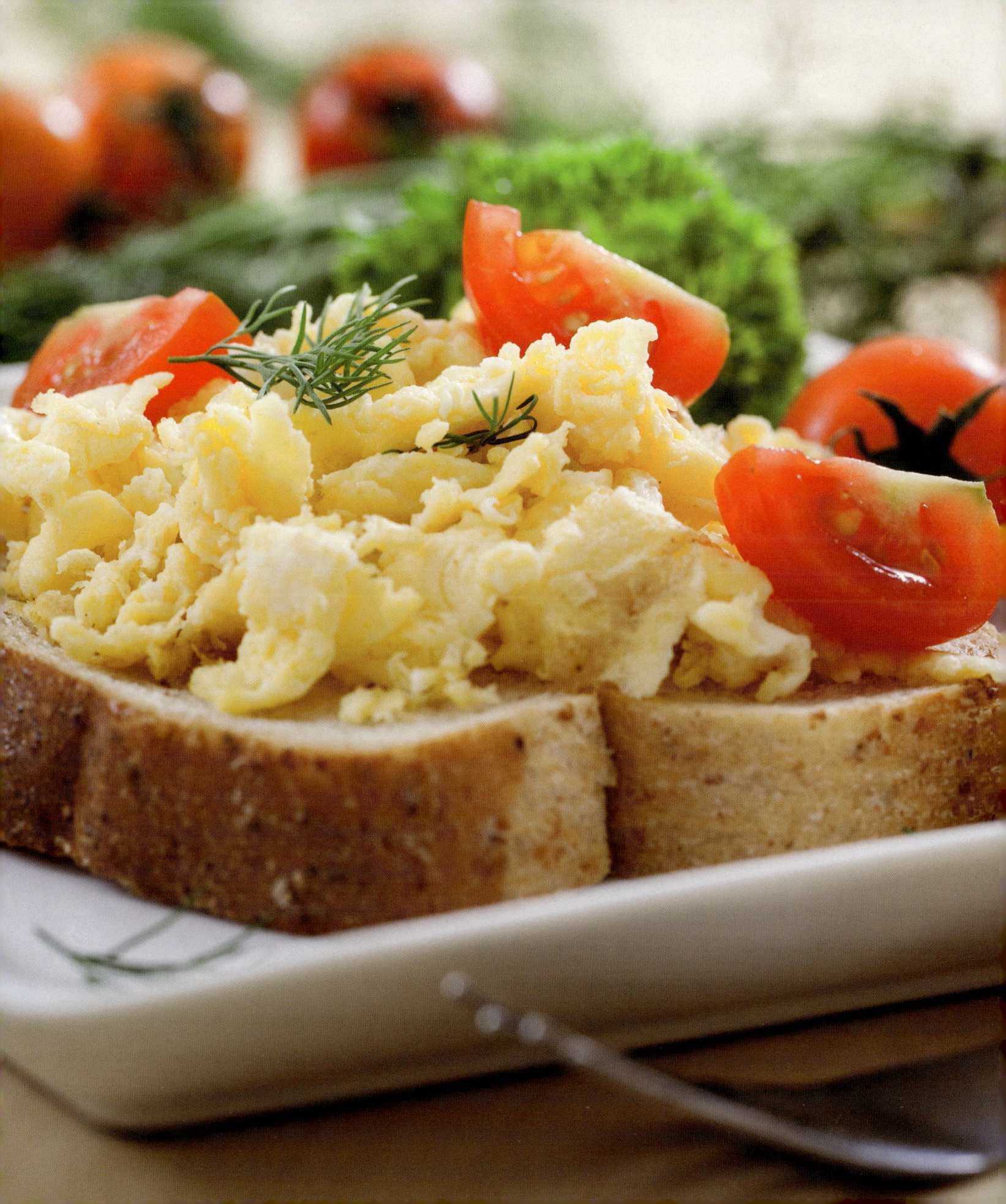

occasional breakfast
bacon & eggs

A favourite for many, keep saturated fat to a minimum by choosing short cut bacon and using a healthy cooking oil such as canola or olive oil.

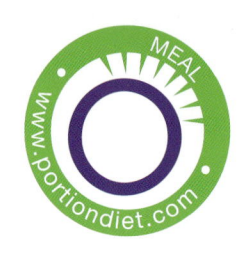

✓ **300 Calories** / 1260 kJ

1 short cut rasher bacon (50 Cals / 210 kJ)
+ 2 fried eggs (160 Cals / 672 kJ)
+ 1 slice toast, no spread (80 Cals / 336 kJ)
+ ½ tomato (<20 Cals / 85 kJ)

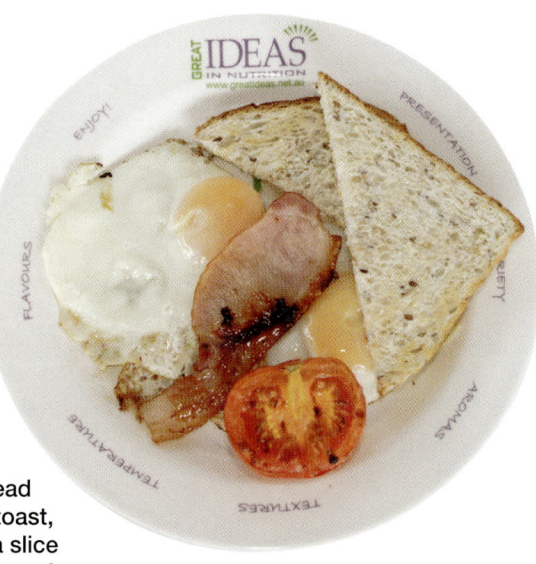

TIP
300/400 Cals – if you'd prefer spread on your toast, swap a slice of bacon for 1½ tsp of spread

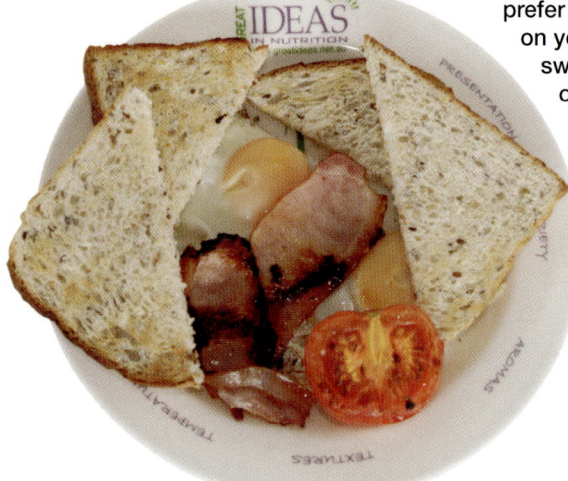

✓ **400 Calories** / 1680 kJ

2 short cut rashers bacon (100 Cals / 420 kJ)
+ 2 eggs (160 Cals / 672 kJ)
+ 2 slices toast, no spread (160 Cals / 672 kJ)
+ ½ tomato (<20 Cals / 85 kJ)

✓ **500 Calories** / 2100 kJ

2 short cut rashers bacon (100 Cals / 420 kJ)
+ 2 eggs (160 Cals / 672 kJ)
+ 2 slices toast (160 Cals / 672 kJ)
+ 3 tsp spread (100 Cals / 420 kJ)
+ ½ tomato (<20 Cals / 85 kJ)

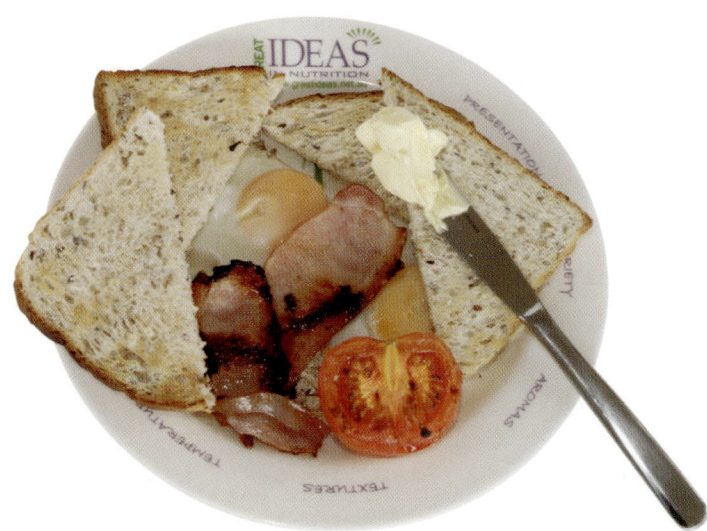

Note: Exact Calories used in the calculation of these meals.

54 | BREAKFAST

occasional breakfast

pancakes

Enjoy your own recipe or try prepared pancake mixes.

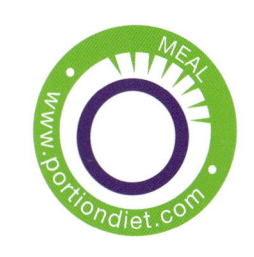

300 Calories / 1260 kJ

2 x 5 in / 13 cm pancakes (160 Cals / 672 kJ)
+ 2 Tbsp maple syrup (140 Cals / 588 kJ)
+ 5 strawberries (<20 Cals / 85 kJ)

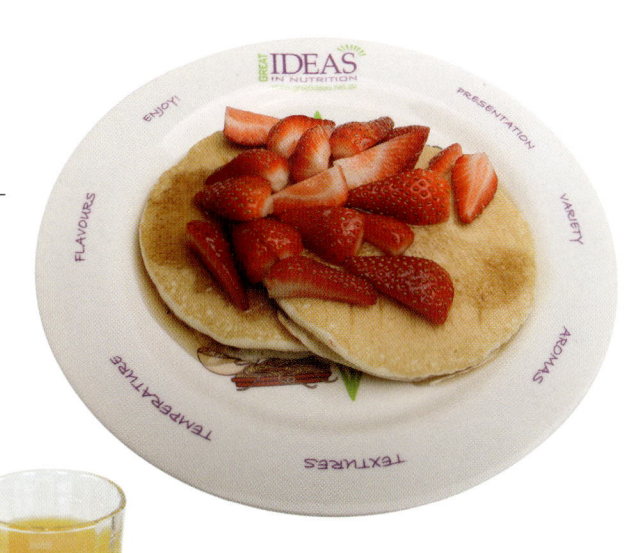

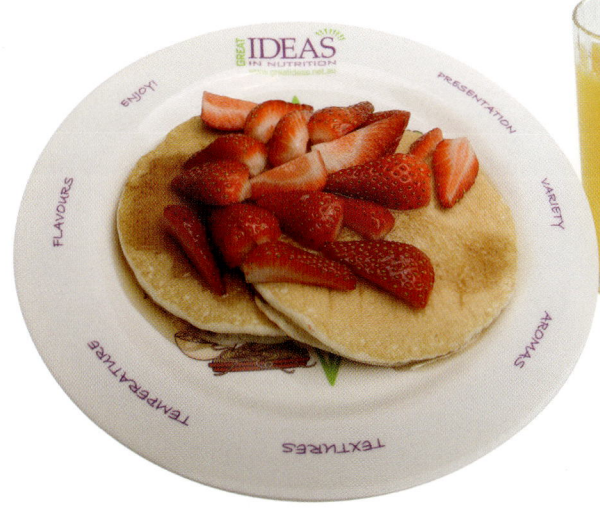

400 Calories / 1680 kJ

2 x 5 in / 13 cm pancakes (160 Cals / 672 kJ)
+ 2 Tbsp maple syrup (140 Cals / 588 kJ)
+ 1 Add On* (6.7 fl oz / 200 ml juice)
(100 Cals / 420 kJ)
+ 5 strawberries (<20 Cals / 85 kJ)

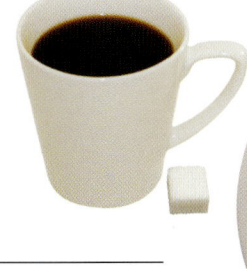

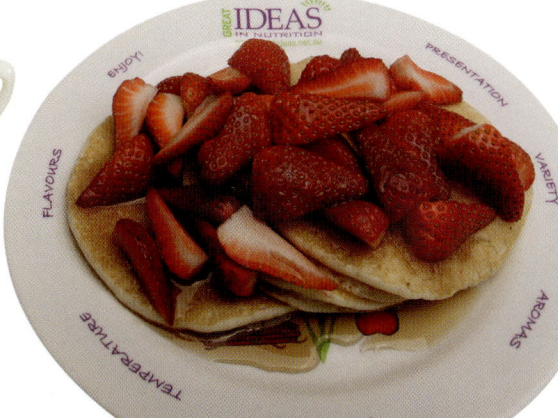

500 Calories / 2100 kJ

3 x 5 in / 13 cm pancakes (240 Cals / 1008 kJ)
+ 3 Tbsp maple syrup (210 Cals / 882 kJ)
+ 5 strawberries (<20 Cals / 85 kJ)
+ tea with 1 tsp sugar (<20 Cals / 85 kJ)

*For Add Ons refer to Appendix 2 on page 132. For Free Foods refer to Appendix 3 on page 134.

BREAKFAST | 55

occasional breakfast

crumpets

Now available in fingers or rounds. 3 fingers = 2 rounds. Aim to limit the use of butter or margarine as it quickly disappears into the holes of the crumpet.

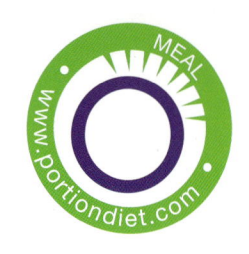

300 Calories / 1260 kJ

3 crumpet fingers (165 Cals / 693 kJ)
+ 2 tsp spread (70 Cals / 294 kJ)
+ 2 tsp honey/syrup (50 Cals / 210 kJ)

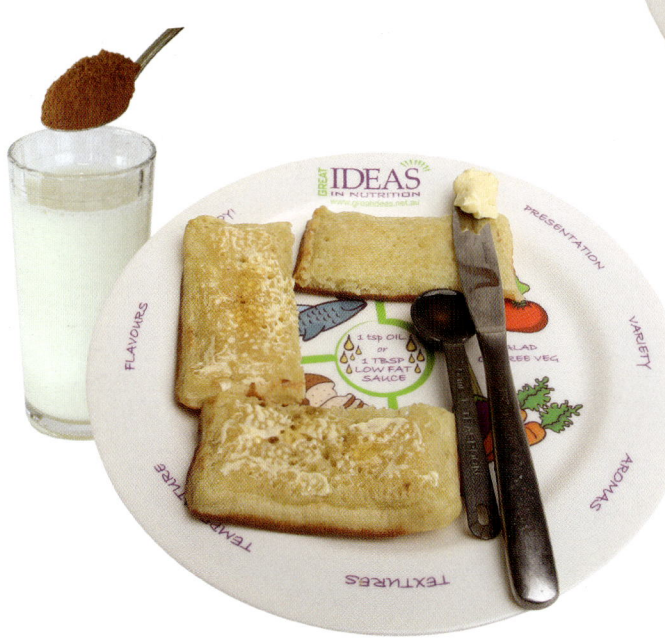

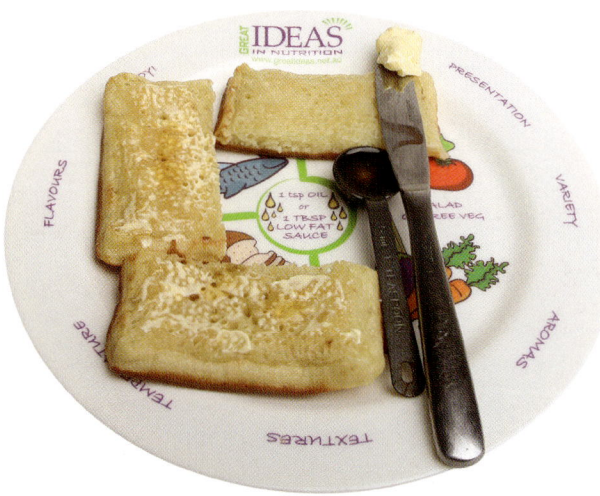

400 Calories / 1680 kJ

3 crumpet fingers (165 Cals / 693 kJ)
+ 2 tsp spread (70 Cals / 294 kJ)
+ 2 tsp honey (50 Cals / 210 kJ)
+ 1 Add On* 6.7 fl oz / 200 ml skim milk (100 Cals / 420 kJ)
+ 1 Free Food – 1 hpd tsp milo (<20 Cals / 85 kJ)

500 Calories / 2100 kJ

4 crumpet fingers (220 Cals / 420 kJ)
+ 2 tsp spread (70 Cals / 294 kJ)
+ 3 tsp honey (75 Cals / 315 kJ)
+ 1 Add On* 6.7 fl oz / 200 ml juice (100 Cals / 420 kJ)

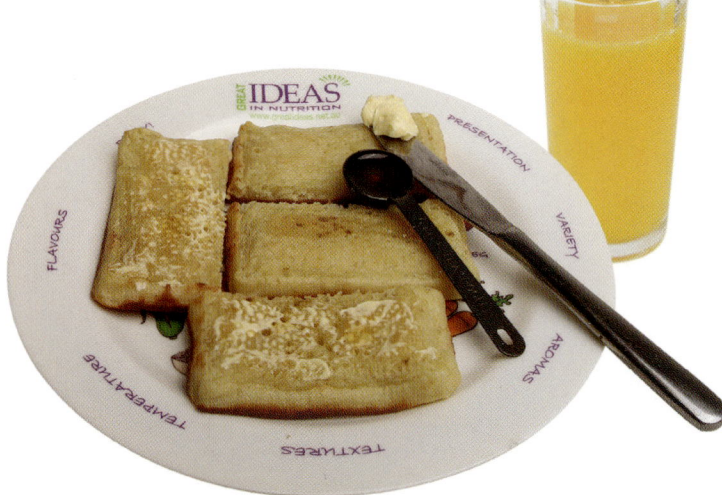

*For Add Ons refer to Appendix 2 on page 132. For Free Foods refer to Appendix 3 on page 134.

56 | BREAKFAST

occasional breakfast

bagels

Bagels are becoming a popular breakfast choice. They are low in fat but are likely to have a higher glycemic index. Enjoy in sweet or savoury combinations by varying Add Ons selections.

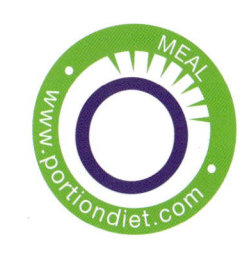

300 Calories / 1260 kJ

1 bagel (250 Cals / 1050 kJ)
+ 2 tsp lite cream cheese (20 Cals / 85 kJ)
+ 2 tsp jam (35 Cals / 147 kJ)

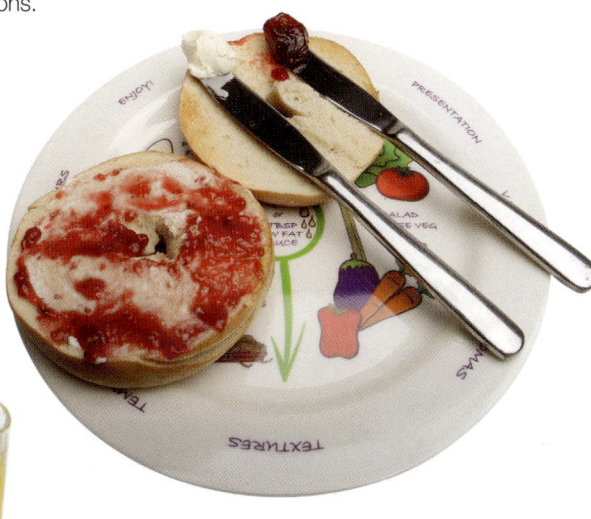

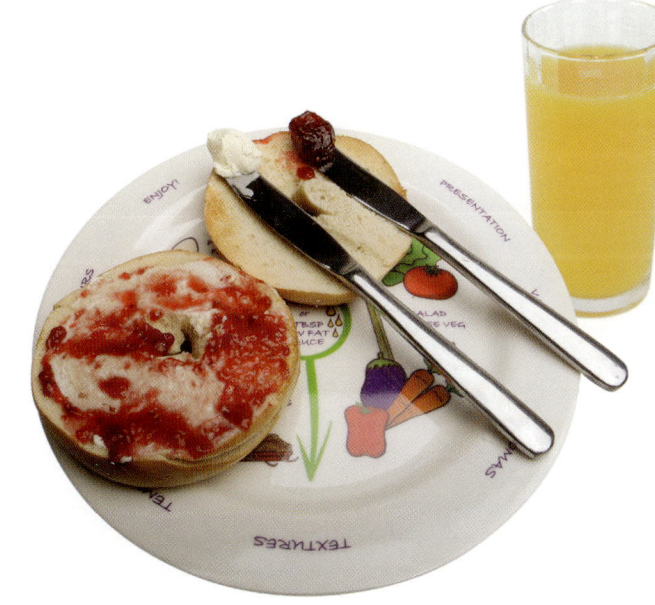

400 Calories / 1680 kJ

1 bagel (250 Cals / 1050 kJ)
+ 2 tsp lite cream cheese (20 Cals / 85 kJ)
+ 2 tsp jam (35 Cals / 147 kJ)
+ 1 Add On* – 6.7 fl oz / 200 ml juice (100 Cals / 420 kJ)

500 Calories / 2100 kJ

1 bagel (250 Cals / 1050 kJ)
+ 2 tsp lite cream cheese (20 Cals / 85 kJ)
+ 2 tsp jam (35 Cals / 147 kJ)
+ 2 Add Ons* – 6.7 fl oz / 200 ml juice (100 Cals / 420 kJ) and 6.7 fl oz / 200 ml skim cappuccino (100 Cals / 420 kJ)

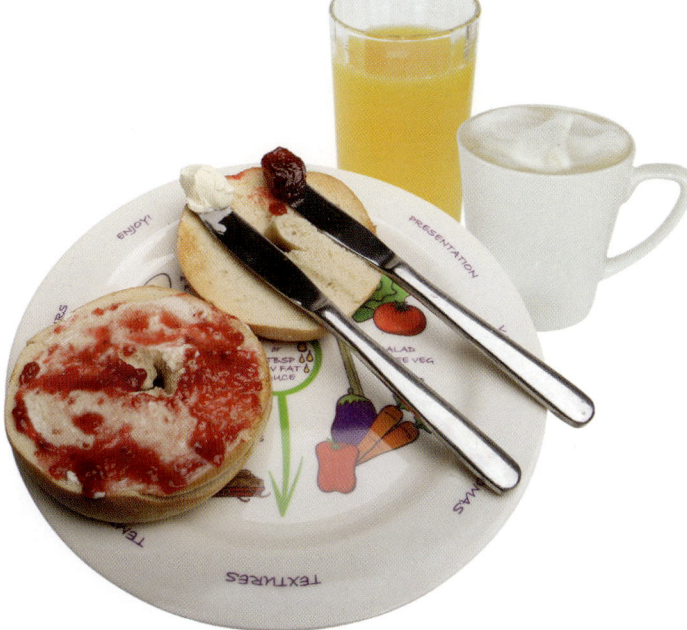

*For Add Ons refer to Appendix 2 on page 132. For Free Foods refer to Appendix 3 on page 134.

BREAKFAST | 57

occasional breakfast

croissant

Croissants come in varying sizes. We've used a 50 g Sara Lee croissant, but be aware that the larger bakery offerings may weigh up to double this. Croissants are also high in saturated fat, so keep it to one.

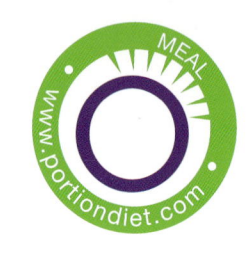

300 Calories / 1260 kJ

1 small croissant (200 Cals / 840 kJ)
+ 2 tsp spread (70 Cals / 294 kJ)
+ 2 tsp jam (35 Cals / 147 kJ)

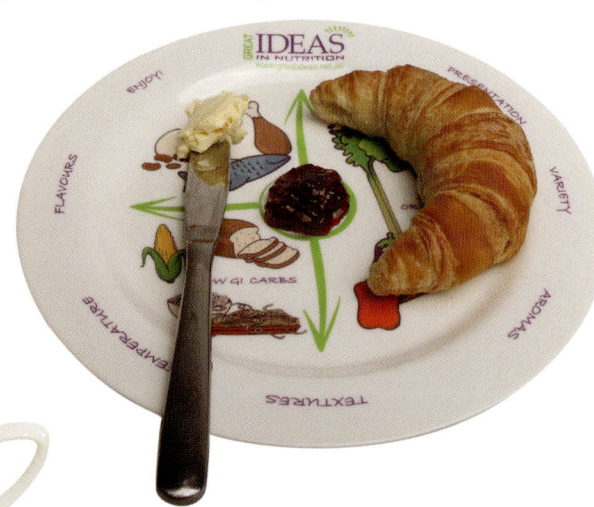

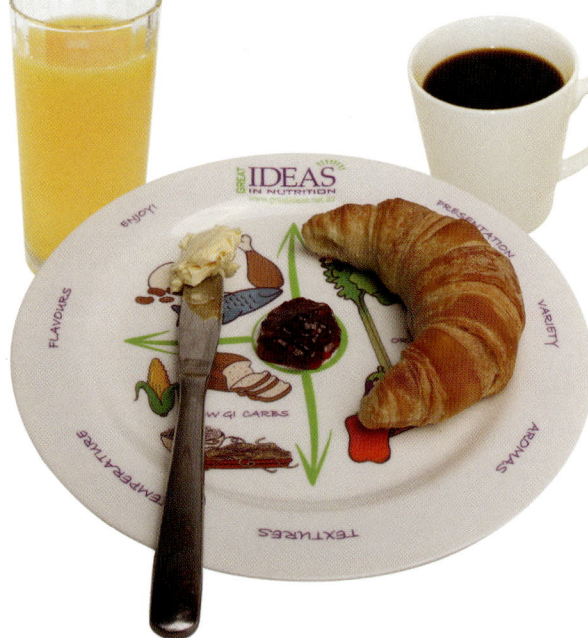

400 Calories / 1680 kJ

1 small croissant (200 Cals / 840 kJ)
+ 2 tsp spread (70 Cals / 294 kJ)
+ 2 tsp jam (35 Cals / 147 kJ)
+ 1 Add On* 6.7 fl oz / 200 ml juice (100 Cals / 420 kJ)
+ 1 Free Food* (tea, <20 Cals / 85 kJ)

500 Calories / 2100 kJ

1 small croissant (200 Cals / 840 kJ)
+ 2 tsp spread (70 Cals / 294 kJ)
+ 2 tsp jam (35 Cals / 147 kJ)
+ 2 Add Ons* – 6.7 fl oz / 200 ml juice (100 Cals / 420 kJ) and 6.7 fl oz / 200 ml skim cappuccino (100 Cals / 420 kJ)

*For Add Ons refer to Appendix 2 on page 132.
For Free Foods refer to Appendix 3 on page 134.

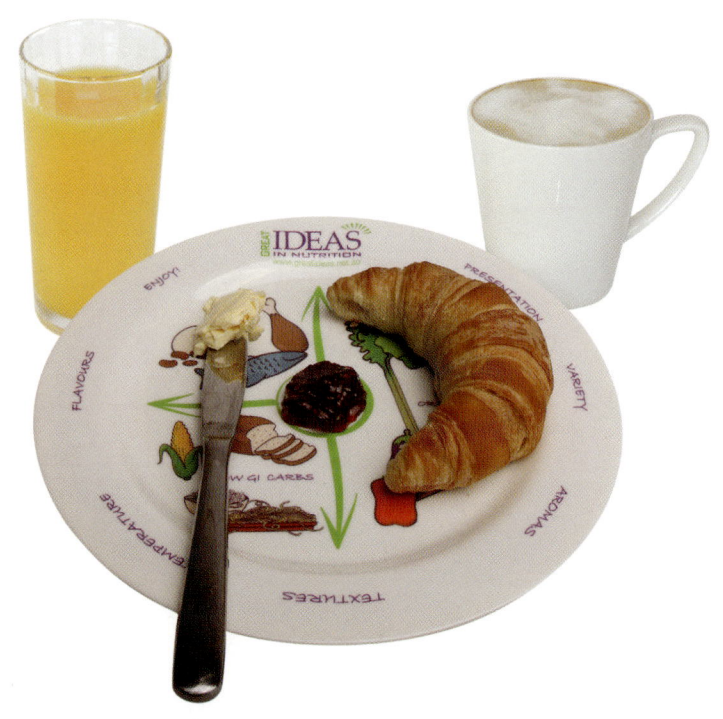

BREAKFAST

occasional breakfast
fast food breakfast

High-fat fast food breakfasts can leave you hungry sooner because as the fat goes up the volume goes down. The specific choice set out below is also high in saturated fat.

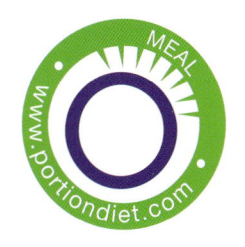

300 Calories / 1260 kJ

1 bacon and egg muffin (300 Cals / 1260 kJ)

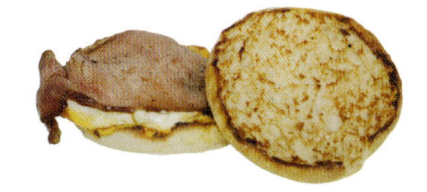

400 Calories / 1680 kJ

1 bacon and egg muffin (300 Cals / 1260 kJ)
+ 1 Add On* 6.7 fl oz / 200 ml juice
(100 Cals / 420 kJ)

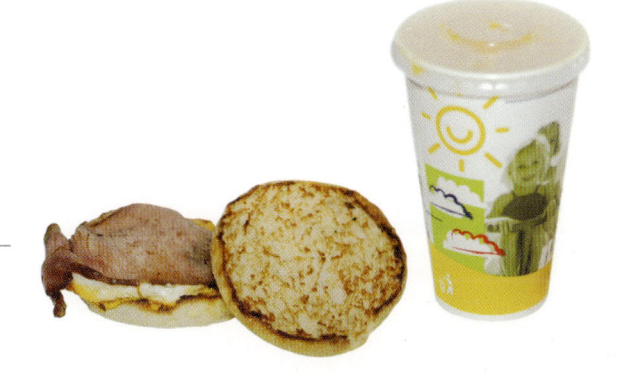

500 Calories / 2100 kJ

1 bacon and egg muffin (300 Cals / 1260 kJ)
+ 1 hash brown (120 Cals / 504 kJ)
+ 1 Add On* 6.7 fl oz / 200 ml juice
(100 Cals / 420 kJ)

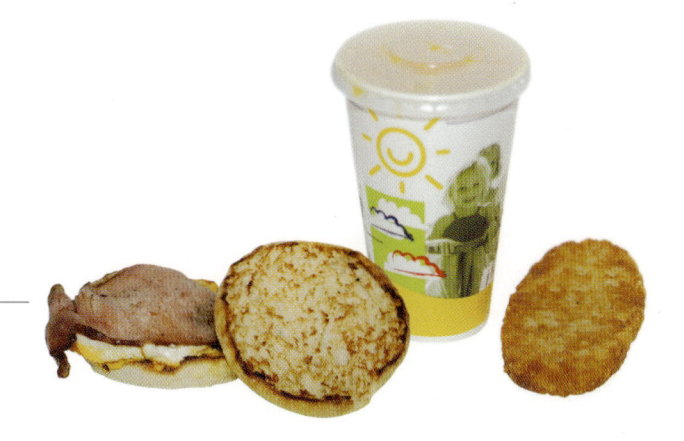

*For Add Ons refer to Appendix 2 on page 132. For Free Foods refer to Appendix 3 on page 134.

occasional breakfast

waffle

We've used frozen waffles, so if you make your own, be guided by the size and suggested weight of approx 1.3 oz / 40 g for one waffle.

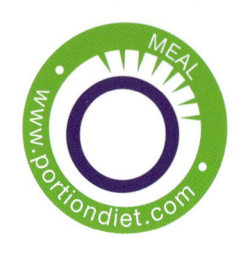

300 Calories / 1260 kJ

1 waffle (140 Cals / 588 kJ)
+ 2 tsp butter (70 Cals / 294 kJ)
+ 4 tsp maple syrup (60 Cals / 240 kJ)

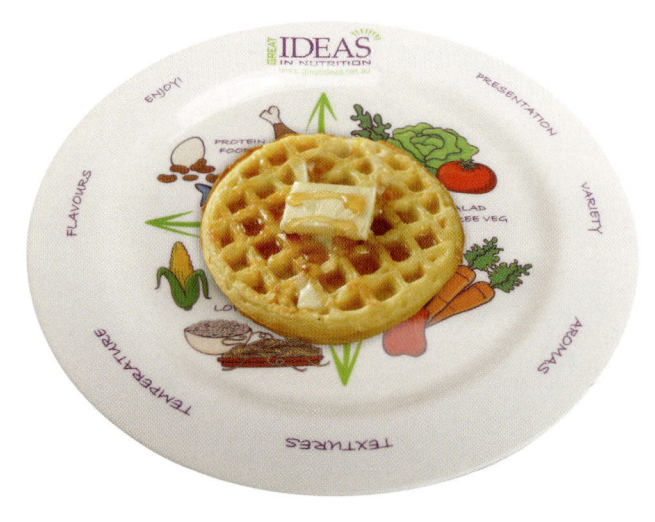

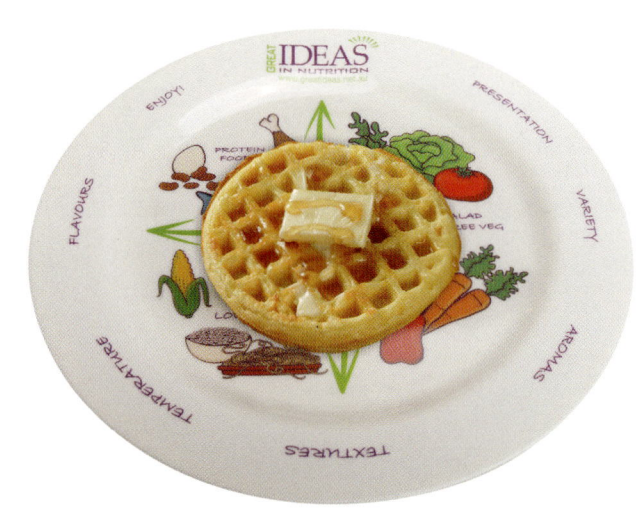

400 Calories / 1680 kJ

1 waffle (140 Cals / 588 kJ)
+ 2 tsp butter (70 Cals / 294 kJ)
+ ¼ cup / 2 fl oz / 60 ml maple syrup (190 Cals / 798 kJ)

500 Calories / 2100 kJ

2 waffles (280 Cals / 1176 kJ)
+ 2 tsp butter (70 Cals / 294 kJ)
+ 1.7 fl oz / 50 ml maple syrup (160 Cals / 672 kJ)

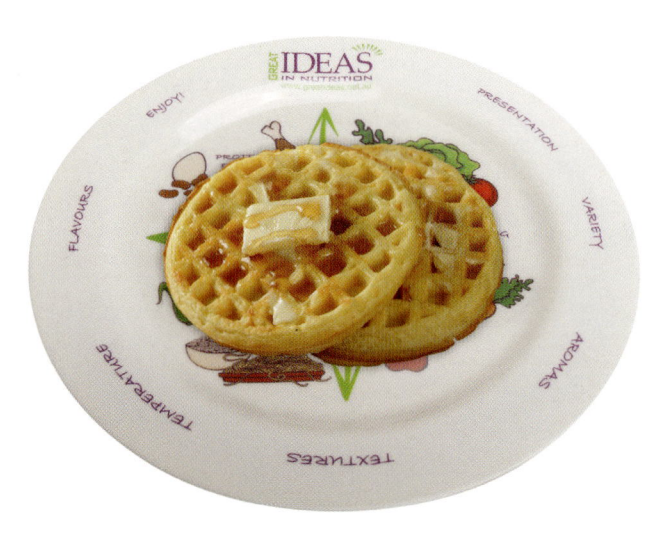

occasional breakfast
donut

Donuts are a very high-fat choice. Keep these for those rare occasions when they seem like a good idea.

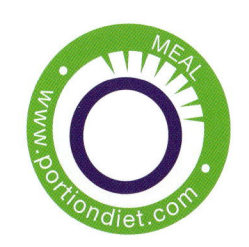

300 Calories / 1260 kJ

1 cinnamon donut (200 Cals / 840 kJ)
+ 6.7 fl oz / 200 ml reduced fat milk
(100 Cals / 420 kJ)

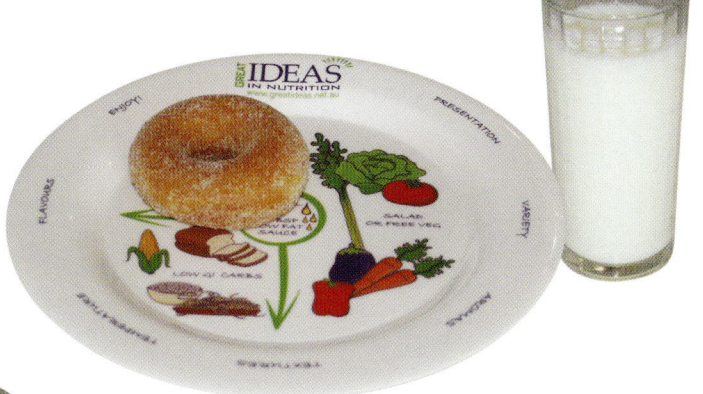

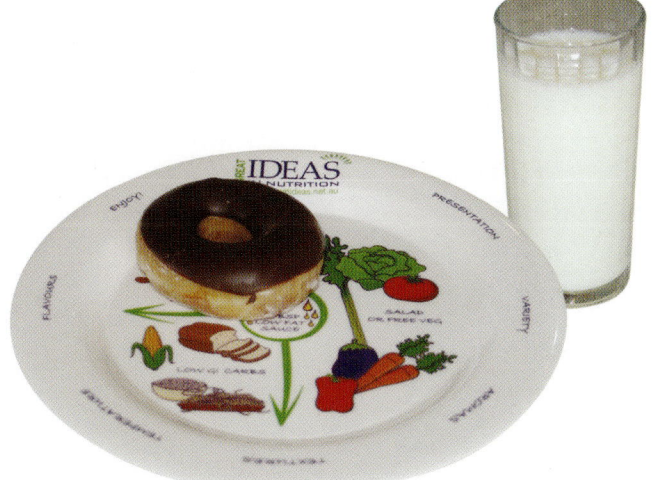

400 Calories / 1680 kJ

1 iced donut (260 Cals / 1092 kJ)
+ 6.7 fl oz / 200 ml reduced fat milk
(100 Cals / 420 kJ)

500 Calories / 2100 kJ

2 cinnamon donuts (400 Cals / 1680 kJ)
+ 6.7 fl oz / 200 ml reduced fat milk
(100 Cals / 420 kJ)

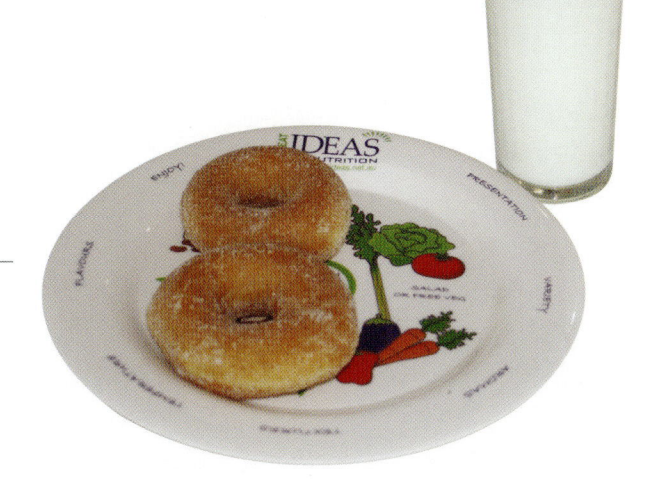

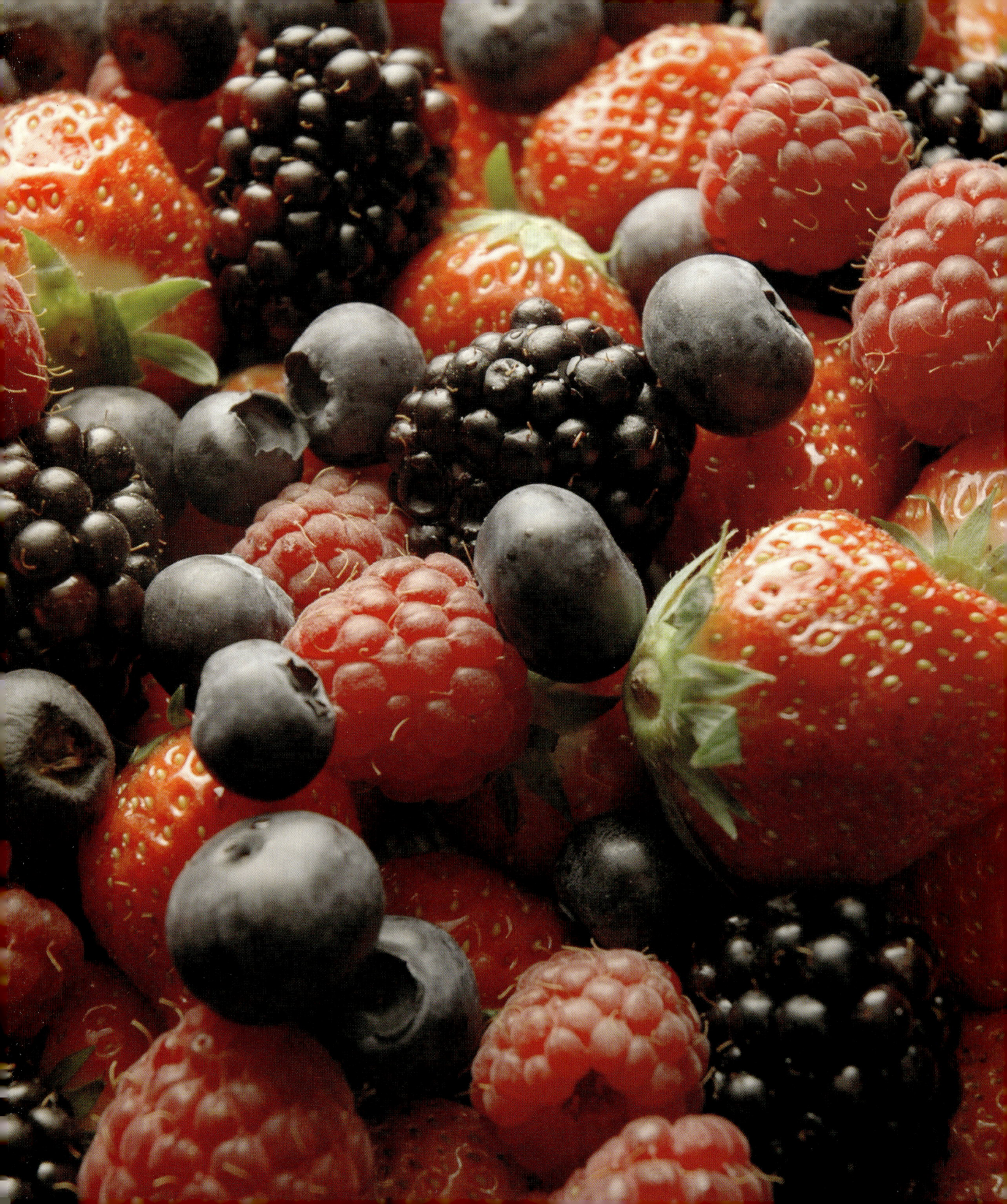

CHAPTER 7

snacks

Snacks are best planned for – make them healthy most of the time. They help control appetite at meal times and keep metabolism clicking over. Choose a morning, afternoon and supper snack according to the colour guide below. Snacks in the everyday section have been assessed against nutritional criteria and are portion controlled at approx. 100 Cals / 420 kJ or 200 Cals / 840 kJ per serve. Occasional snacks also taste great but are either likely to have a higher GI, a high saturated fat content or don't meet nutritional criteria. Use them within your occasional choices limit (see page 28). For nutritional balance, focus snacks around fruit, dairy and nuts.

Everyday 100 Calorie / 420 kJ snack menu*

Fruit.................................. 65
Vegetables & dip.............. 66
Dairy................................. 68
Frozen desserts............... 71
Nuts & seeds................... 72
Bars 74
Biscuits & crackers.......... 75
Miscellaneous.................. 76

Occasional 100 Calorie / 420 kJ snack menu

Dairy................................. 79
Biscuits & crackers.......... 80
Cakes & desserts............ 81
Chocolates & lollies......... 82
Bars 84
Miscellaneous.................. 85
Alcohol 86

200 Calorie / 420 kJ snack menu*

Everyday 88
Occasional 90

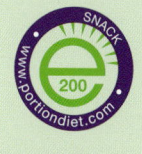

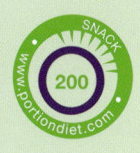

* All snacks selected for the 100 Cal / 420 kJ section contain 60–130 Cals / 252–546 kJ. Snacks selected for the 200 Cal / 840 kJ section contain 160–230 Cals / 672–966 kJ.

200 Cal / 840 kJ snacks can easily be devised by doubling the options shown above.
A few additional items that are portion controlled at 200 Calories / 840 kJ are shown here also.

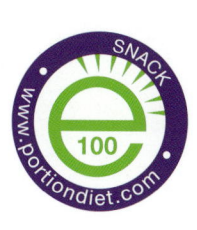

Snack guide
✓ 3 x 100 Cal / 420 kJ snacks / day
✓ 3 x 100 Cal / 420 kJ snacks / day
✓ 2 x 200 Cal / 840 kJ snacks / day **and** 1 x 100 Cal / 420 kJ snacks / day
✓ 3 x 200 Cal / 840 kJ snacks / day

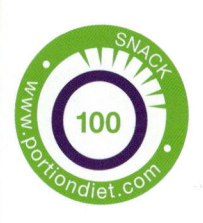

Add your own favourites by calculating the appropriate serve from Allan Borushek's *The CalorieKing Calorie, Fat and Carbohydrate Counter* or apps CalorieKing or My Fitness Pal.

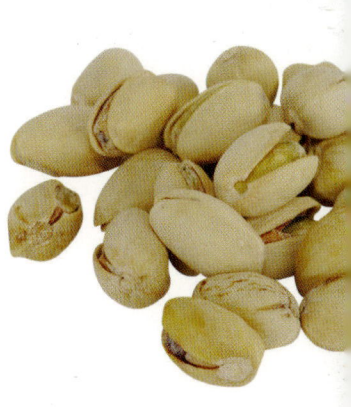

SNACKS | 63

"I think most people would like
to eat the right amount,
if only they knew what that was."

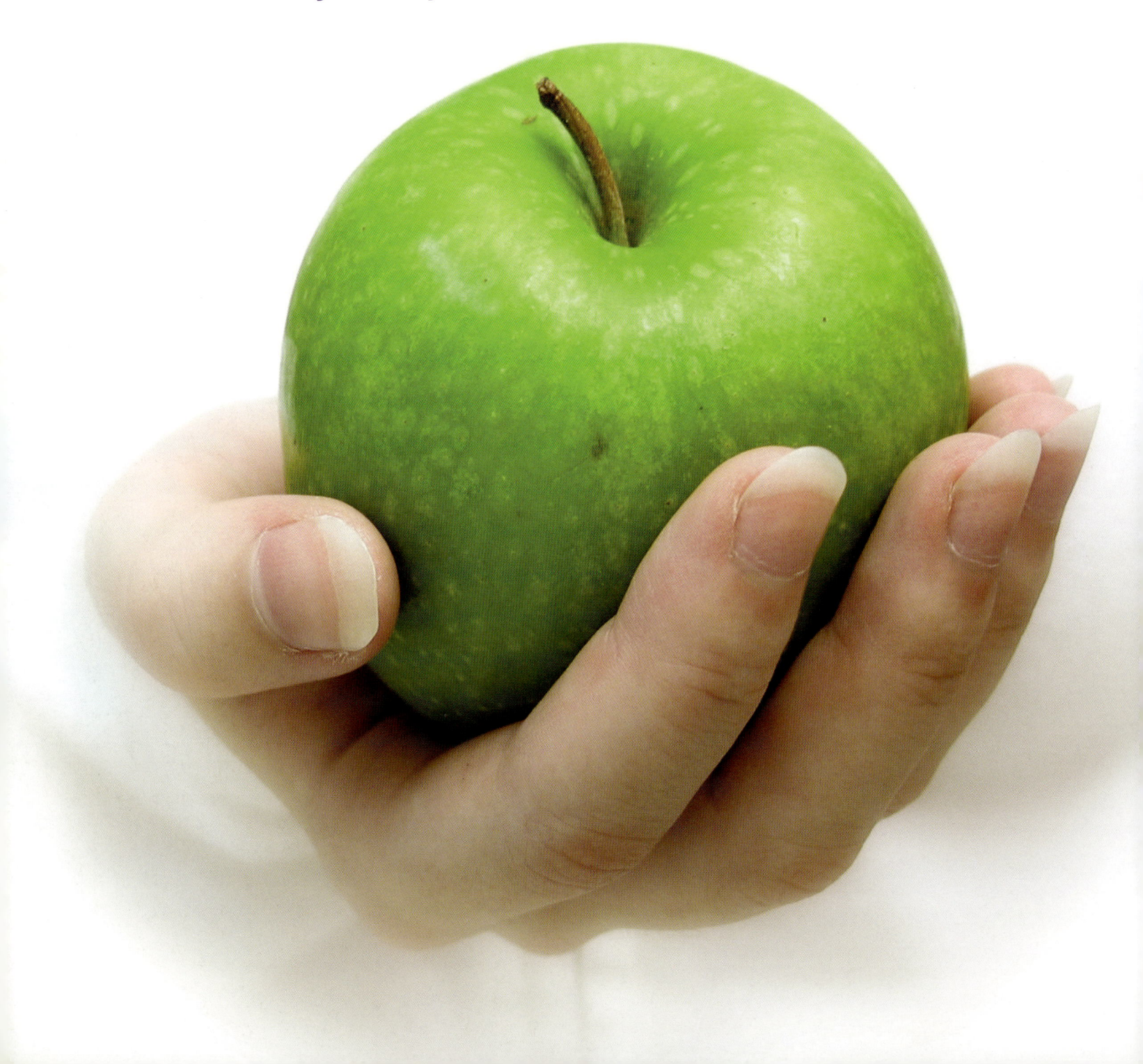

everyday snacks

fruit

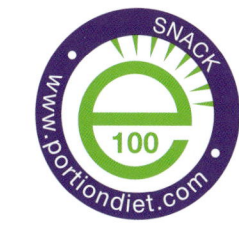

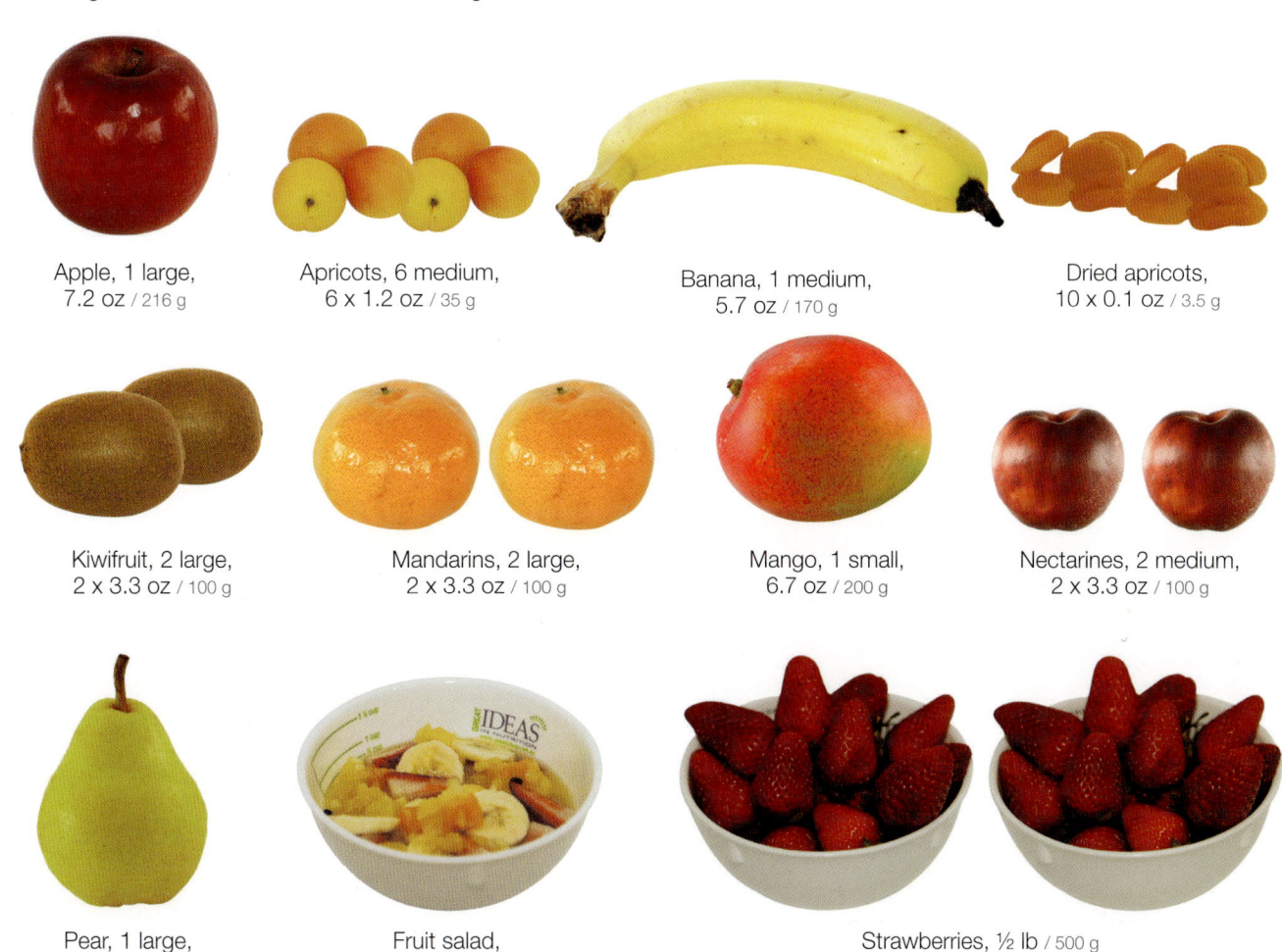

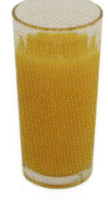

Fruit is a perfect portion controlled snack. A 100 Cal / 420 kJ fruit snack consists of 2 small fruit serves (see Appendix 1) or 1 large fruit serve such as a banana or mango.

Apple, 1 large, 7.2 oz / 216 g

Apricots, 6 medium, 6 x 1.2 oz / 35 g

Banana, 1 medium, 5.7 oz / 170 g

Dried apricots, 10 x 0.1 oz / 3.5 g

Kiwifruit, 2 large, 2 x 3.3 oz / 100 g

Mandarins, 2 large, 2 x 3.3 oz / 100 g

Mango, 1 small, 6.7 oz / 200 g

Nectarines, 2 medium, 2 x 3.3 oz / 100 g

Pear, 1 large, 6.7 oz / 200 g

Fruit salad, 1 cup

Strawberries, ½ lb / 500 g

Various brands, Fruit juice, 6.7-8.3 fl oz / 200-250 ml

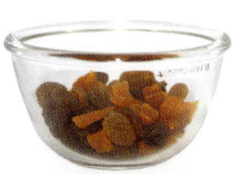

Dried fruit, 2 Tbsp, 1.3 oz / 40 g

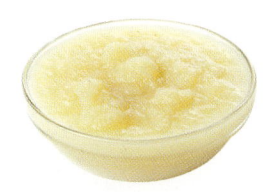

Applesauce, ½ cup, 4.7 oz / 140 g

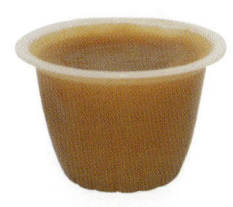

Fruit puree, ½ cup, 4.3 oz / 130 g

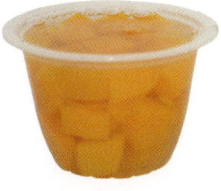

Canned fruit, ½ cup, 4.7 oz / 140 g

TIP Refer to Appendix 1 for more ideas.

everyday snacks
vegetables & dip
Choose one vegetable serve and 1 dip portion.

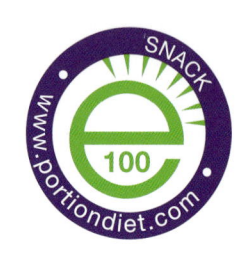

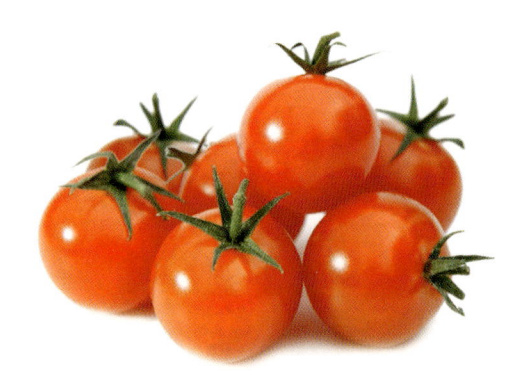

Cherry tomatoes, 7

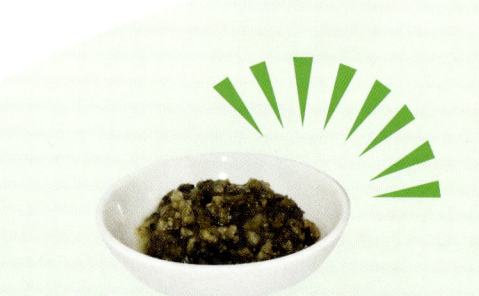

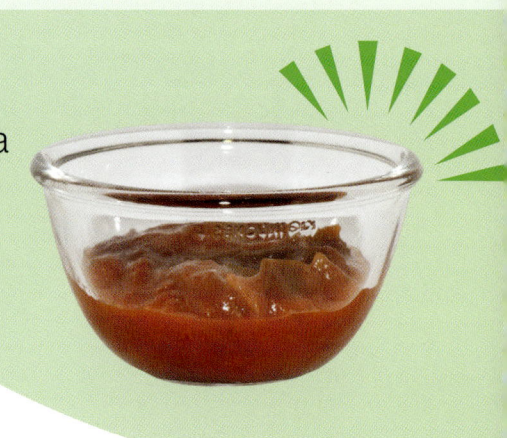

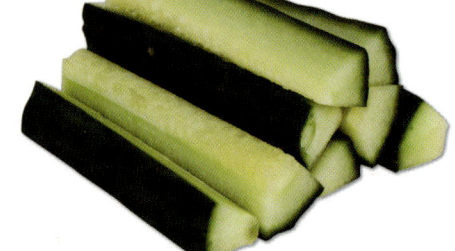

Carrot, 2 oz / 60 g

Cucumber, 5 oz / 150 g

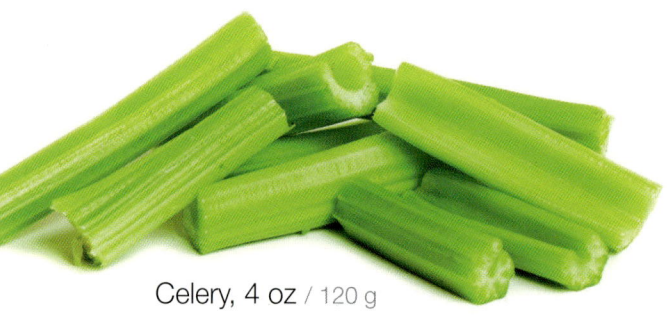

Celery, 4 oz / 120 g

1 Tbsp oily dip or pesto

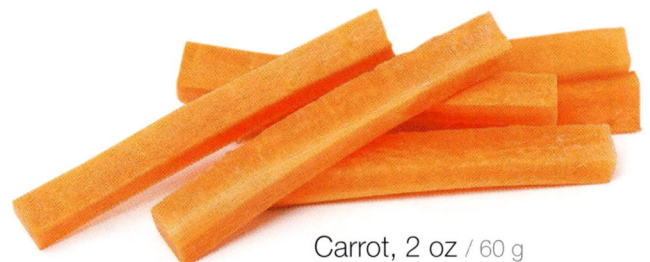

¼ cup salsa or tzatziki

everyday snacks
vegetables & dip *continued*

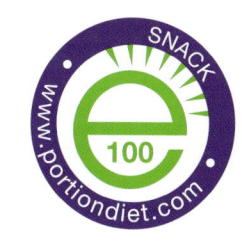

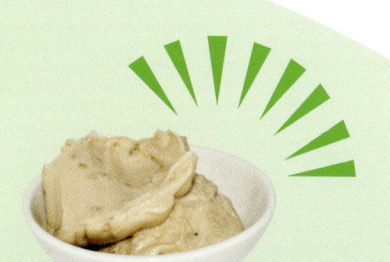

2 Tbsp creamy dip, hommous, guacamole or reduced fat cream cheese

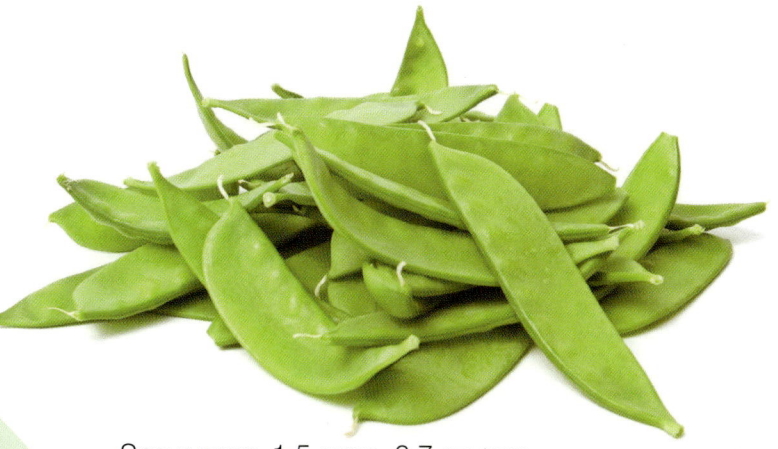

Snow peas, 1.5 cups, 6.7 oz / 200 g

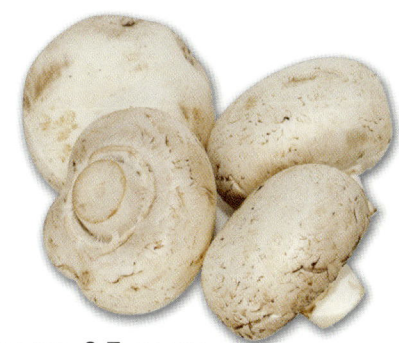

Mushrooms, 2.7 oz / 80 g

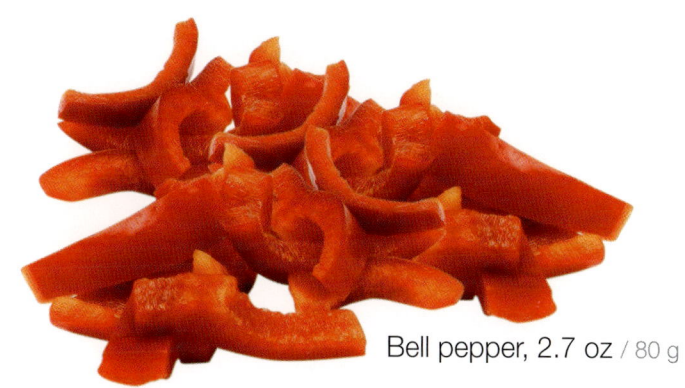

Bell pepper, 2.7 oz / 80 g

Fresh peas or edamame beans, 1 cup in shell, 4.2 oz / 125 g

SNACKS | 67

everyday snacks

dairy

Dairy snacks are a great idea for between meals because the protein keeps you feeling satisfied. Most low fat dairy snacks are low GI despite added sugar.

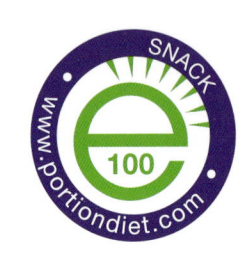

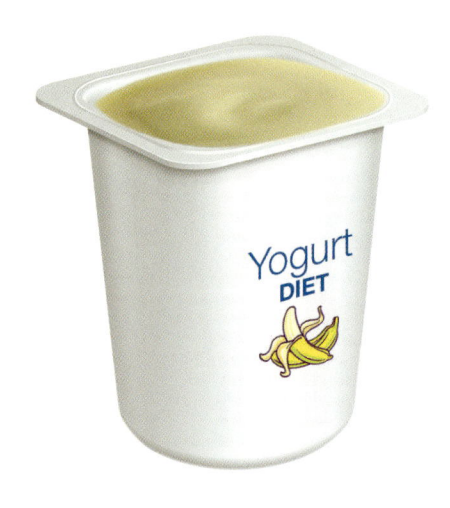

Yoghurt, diet or low fat, natural,*
6.7 oz / 200 g

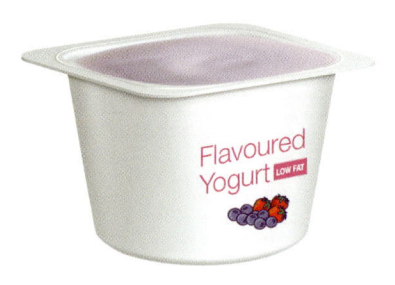

Yoghurt, regular or low fat, flavoured,
3.3 oz / 100 g

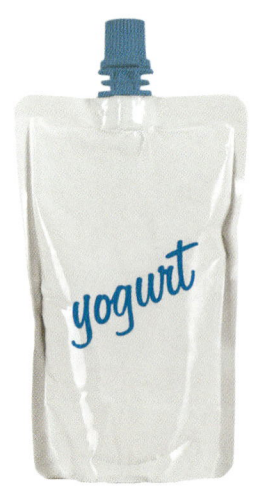

Yoghurt pouch or tube,
2.3 oz / 70 g

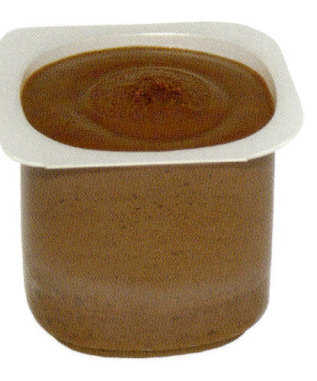

Low fat custard or mousse,
½ cup, 3.3 oz / 100 g

*Diet yoghurt is low fat and artificially sweetened.

everyday snacks
dairy *continued*

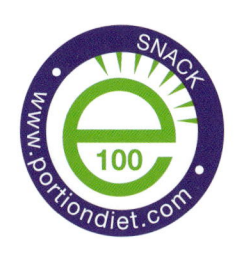

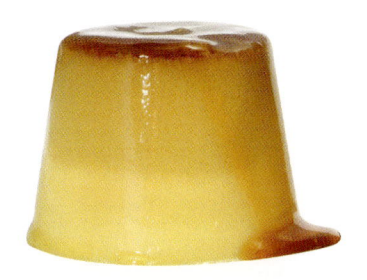

Creme caramel / Spanish style custard,
½ cup, 4 oz / 125 g

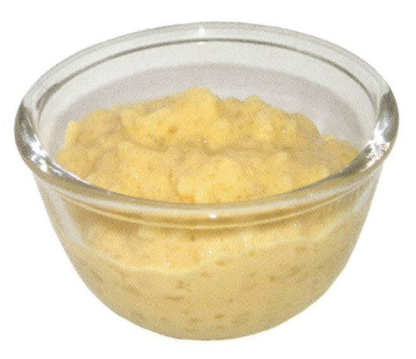

Low fat or sugar free pudding,
½ cup, 4 oz / 125 g

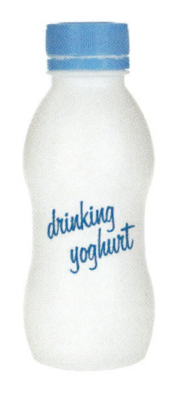

Drinking yoghurt,
3.3 fl oz / 100 ml

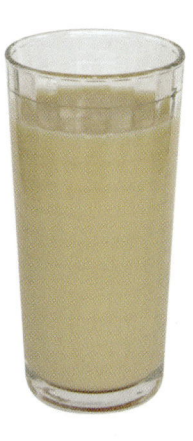

Reduced / low fat / skim milk,
6.7 fl oz / 200 ml

everyday snacks
dairy continued

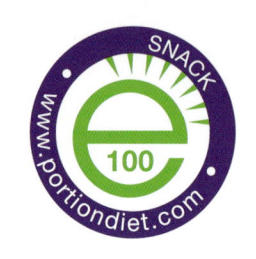

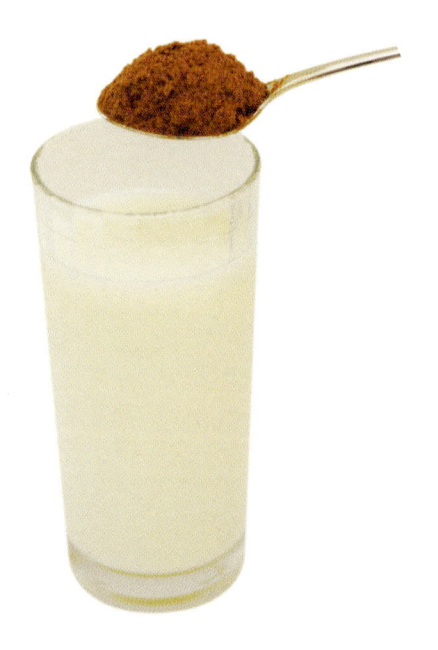

Skim milk, 6.7 fl oz / 200 ml + 1 hpd tsp Milo

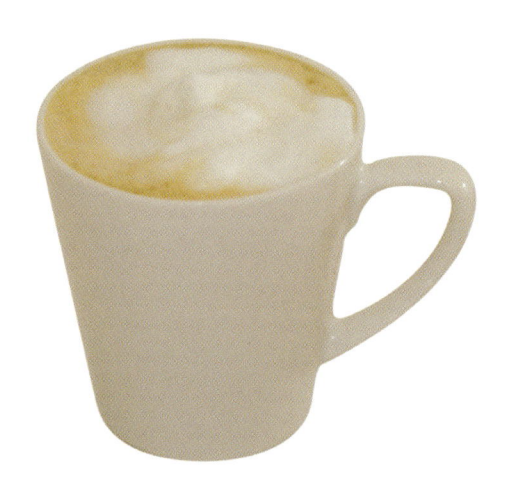

Skinny cappuccino or latte, 6.7 fl oz / 200 ml

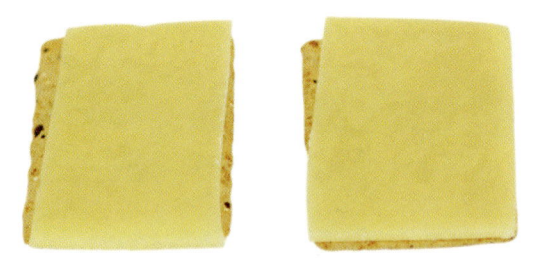

Wholegrain crackers,
2 + 50% reduced fat cheese, 1 slice

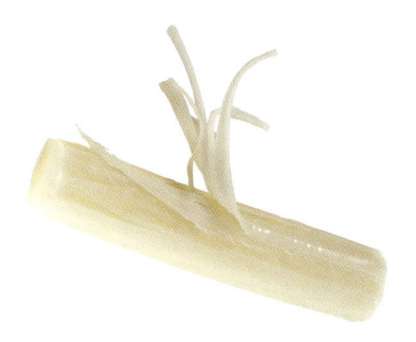

String cheese, 2%, 1 stick

See the Healthy Snack Bible for your local guide to brand named products that fit these criteria.

* Everyday criteria for milk, yoghurts + desserts per 100 Cal / 420 kJ **pack**
  1. 3 g or less of fat
  2. Low GI or 20 g or less of sugar (most dairy foods are low GI)

* Everyday criteria for cheeses per 100 Cal / 420 kJ **serve**
  1. 6g or less of fat

everyday snacks
frozen desserts

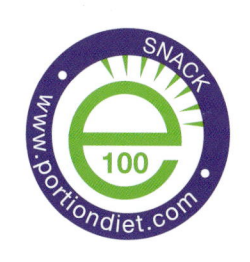

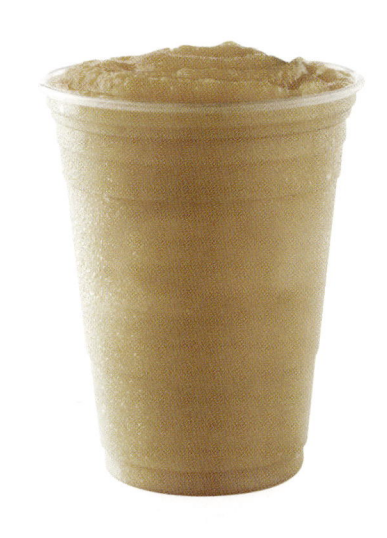

Frappucino coffee flavour, no cream, 12 fl oz / 350 ml

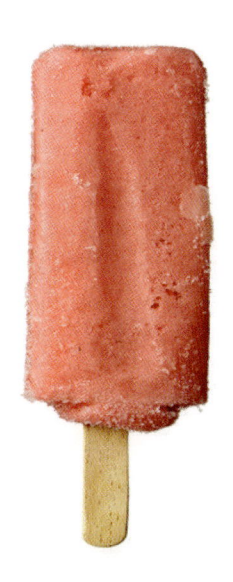

Milk ice, 2 oz / 60 g

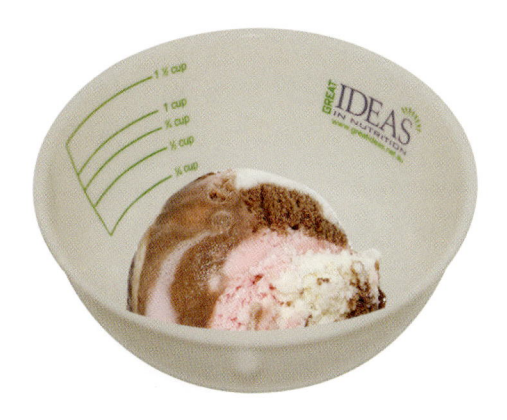

Light ice cream, various brands, 1 scoop, 3.3 fl oz / 100 ml

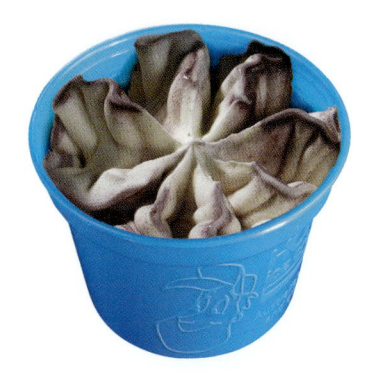

Frozen yoghurt, 1 scoop, 1.5 oz / 45 g

everyday snacks
Nuts & seeds

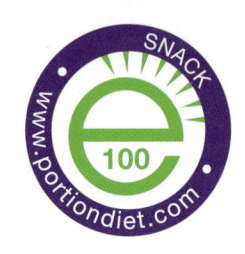

Nuts are a natural and healthy snack. Choose raw and unsalted nuts as the ultimate healthy snack. Just get the portion size right. Nuts may be a perfect, quick and simple solution to the snack times when you are not looking for bulk.

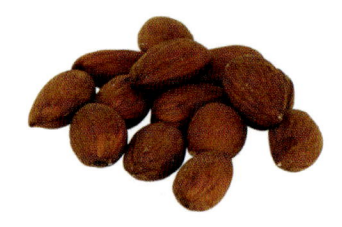

Almonds, 14,
0.7 oz / 20 g

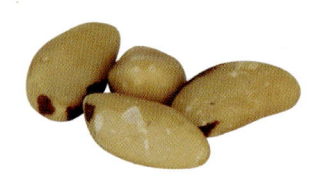

Brazil nuts, 4,
0.7 oz / 20 g

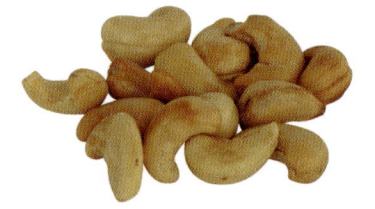

Cashews, 14,
0.7 oz / 20 g

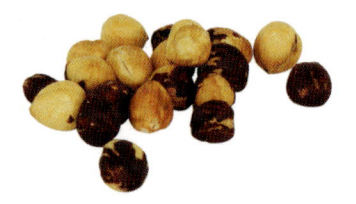

Hazelnuts, 20,
0.5 oz / 15 g

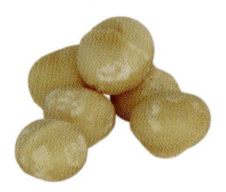

Macadamias, 6,
0.7 oz / 20 g

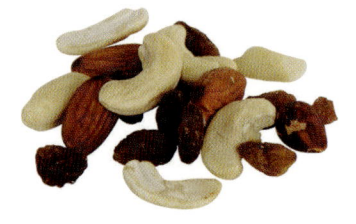

Mixed fruit & nuts,
0.7 oz / 20 g

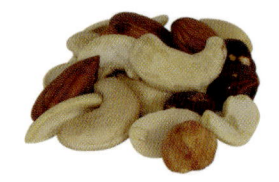

Mixed nuts,
0.7 oz / 18 g

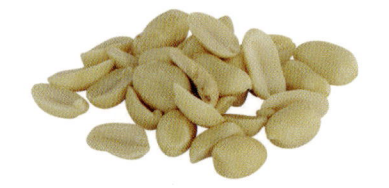

Peanuts, 36 halves,
0.7 oz / 18 g

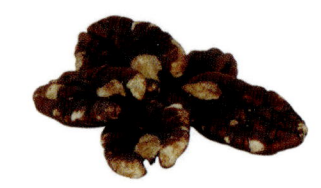

Pecans, 5,
0.7 oz / 20 g

72 | SNACKS

everyday snacks

Nuts & seeds *continued*

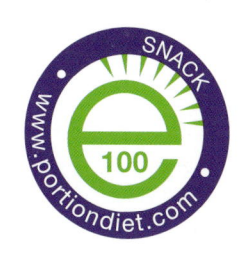

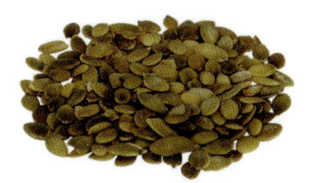

Pepitas, 2 Tbsp,
0.7 oz / 20 g

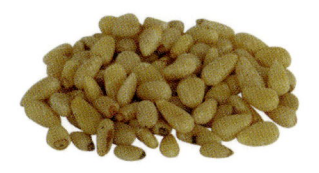

Pinenuts, 2 Tbsp,
0.7 oz / 18 g

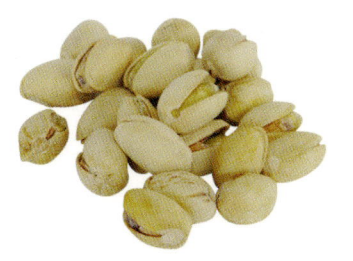

Pistachios, 25,
0.7 oz / 20 g shelled

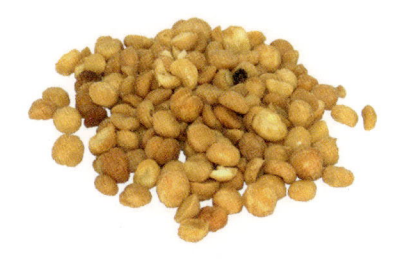

Roasted chickpeas, ¼ cup,
0.8 oz / 25 g

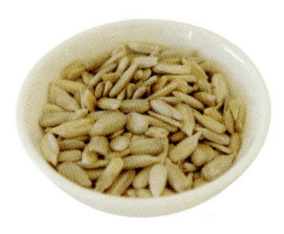

Sunflower seeds, 1.5 Tbsp,
0.7 oz / 18 g

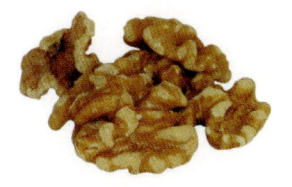

Walnuts, 6,
0.7 oz / 20 g

TIP

You'll note that most serves here are around 20 g, which is roughly the amount that fits into a cupped palm.

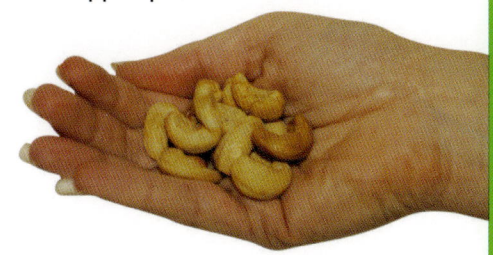

everyday snacks

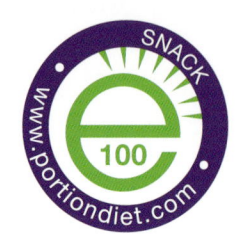

bars

Muesli and fruit bars are a really handy snack to take out with you. They don't require refrigeration, generally don't make a mess, and they can be eaten without having to handle the food. Look for bars with approx 100 Cals / 420 kJ per bar. In general these will weigh 0.7-1 oz / 20 - 30 g. Then check against the nutritional criteria below to determine whether they're healthy enough to eat every day or just occasionally.

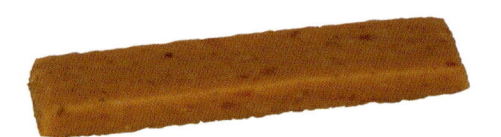

Fruit bar, 0.7 oz / 20 g

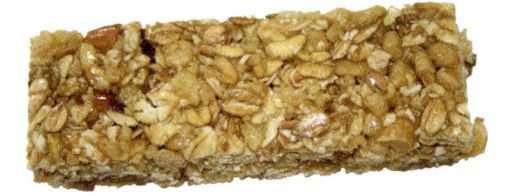

Granola bar, 1 oz / 35 g

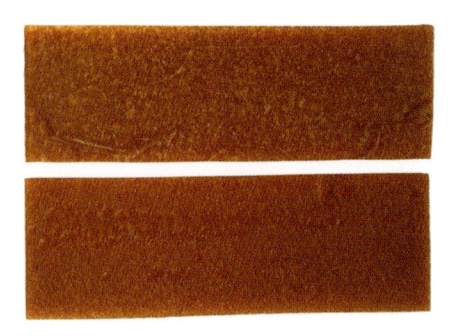

Fruit straps, 2

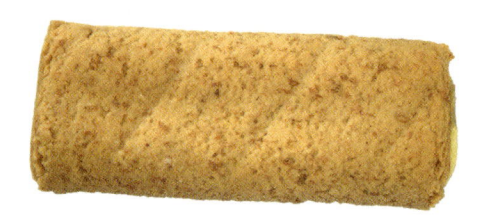

Baked Fruit Bar, 1.3 oz / 40 g

---

*Everyday bar criteria

Approx 100 Cals / 420 kJ per serve and 3 out of 4 of the following criteria:

1. 1 g or more of fibre
2. Low GI or 5 g or less of sugar if no/ little fruit or 15 g or less sugar with significant fruit*
3. 3.5 g or less fat if no nuts or 7.5 g or less fat with nuts.
4. 1 g or less saturated fat.

*Significant fruit is considered to be 25% or more.

SNACKS

everyday snacks

biscuits, cookies & crackers

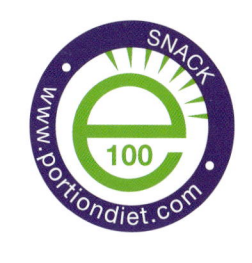

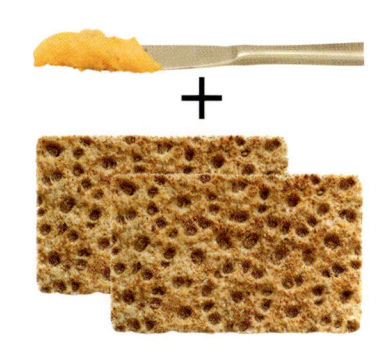

Most biscuits and crackers are high GI however those with either wholegrains or fruit tend to be lower. Try low fat dips with healthy crackers.

Low GI or grainy crackers, 2 large, + 2 tsp low fat dip

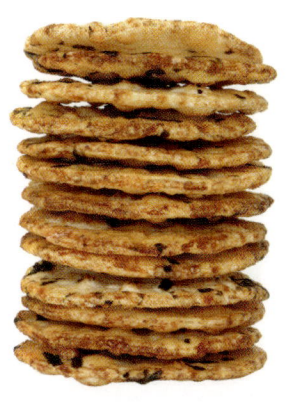

Wholegrain rice crackers, 13

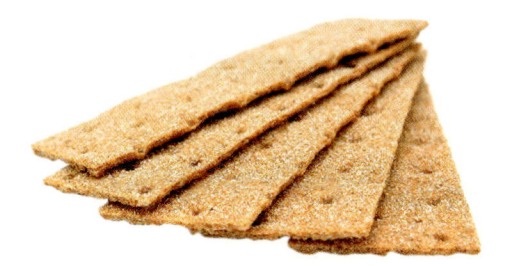

Thin rye crispread, 5, 0.8 oz / 25 g

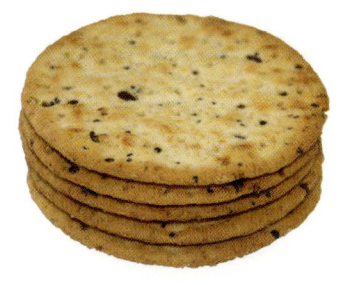

Low GI or grainy crackers, 5 small

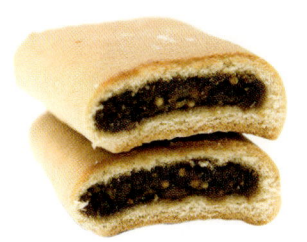

Fruit filled cookies, 2

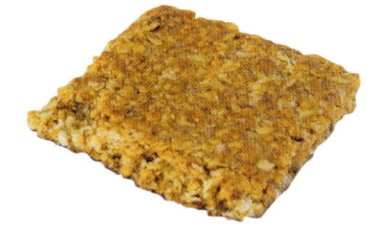

Muesli cookie, 1, 0.5 oz / 17 g

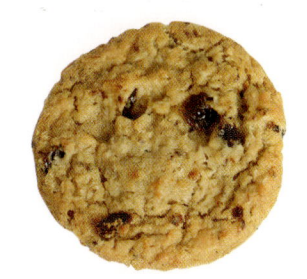

Raisin or oat cookie, 1 standard size, 0.8 oz / 25 g

---

*Everyday biscuit criteria per 100 Cal / 420 kJ serve
1. 3 g or less of saturated fat
2. 200 mg or less of sodium
3. Low GI, or 10% wholegrains or 25% or more of fruit

* Biscuits should meet all criteria. Some products in this category do not declare data relevant to criteria 3, so some professional judgements have been made.

SNACKS | 75

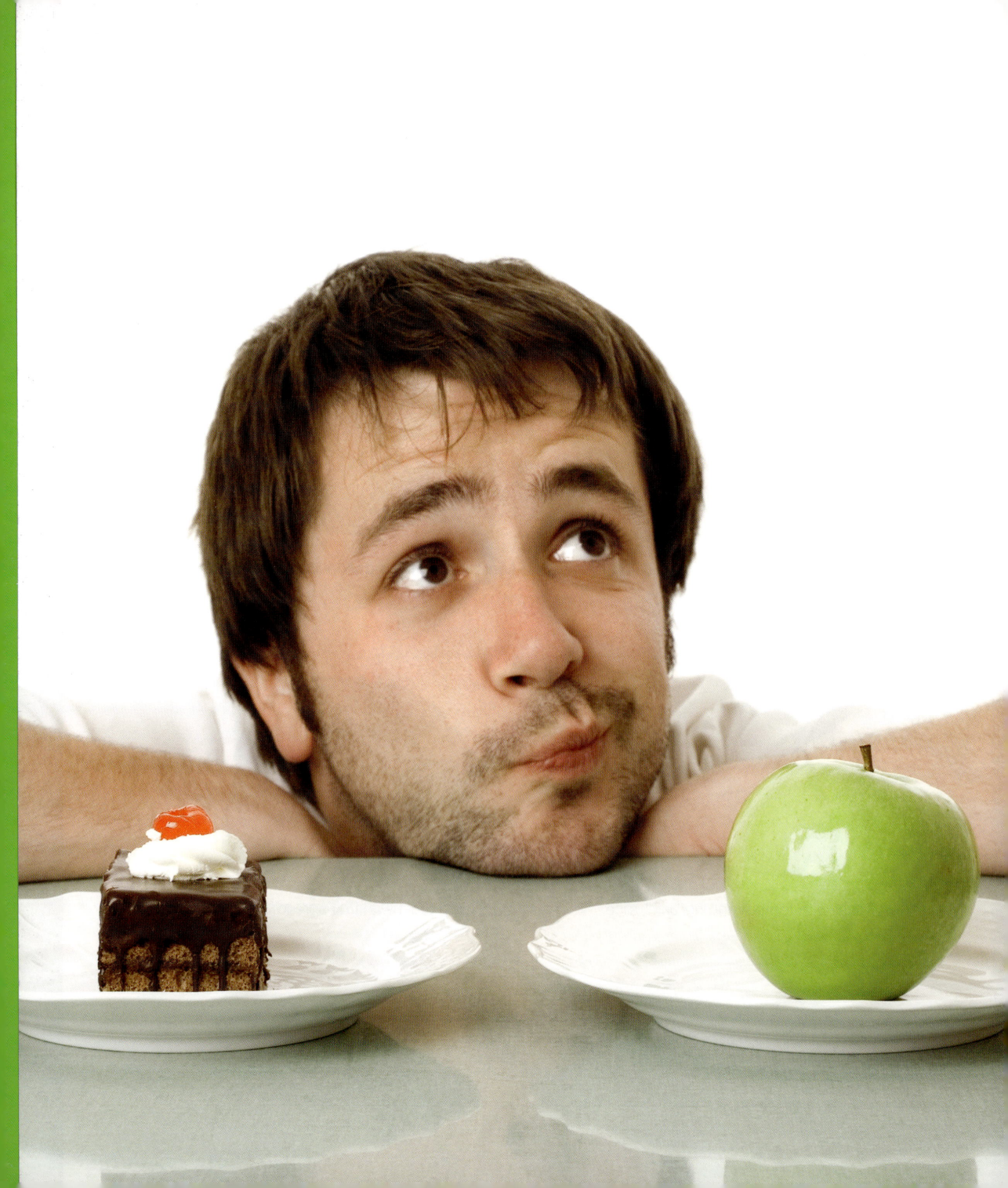

occasional snacks

Occasional snacks are portion controlled and may contain some healthy ingredients known to be higher GI, such as rice, or may be designed for a pure taste experience. Enjoy them occasionally the way they were intended. No guilt required. Remember to eat them slowly and enjoy every morsel, and when they're gone, they're gone.

dairy

1 cheese slice, 0.7 oz / 20 g

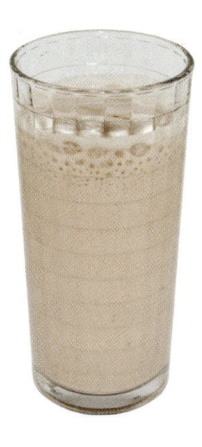

Whole milk milkshake, 6.7 fl oz / 200 ml

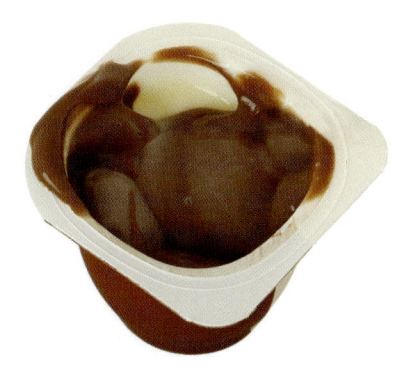

Chocolate custard, ½ cup

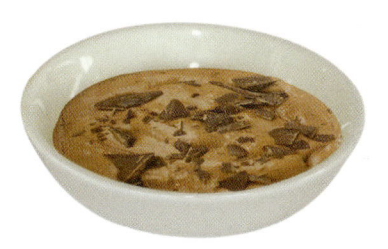

Rich dairy dessert, ¼ cup

occasional snacks
biscuits & crackers

Enjoy higher GI crackers with low fat dip occasionally.

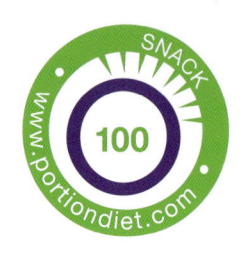

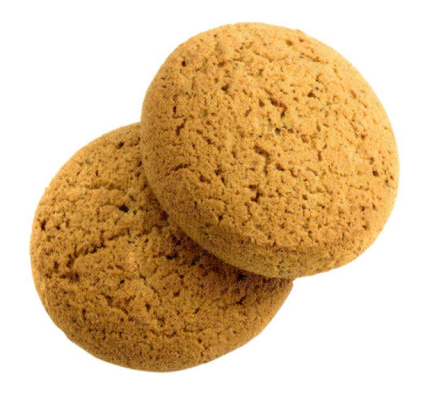

2 plain sweet cookies / biscuits, 0.8 oz / 25 g

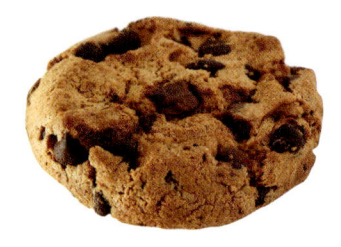

1 premium choc chip or homemade small

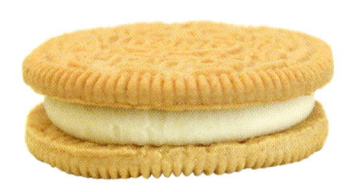

1 cream cookie / biscuit, 0.6 oz / 18 g

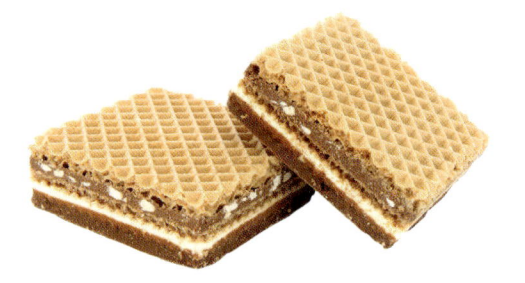

2 cream wafers, 0.5 oz / 15 g

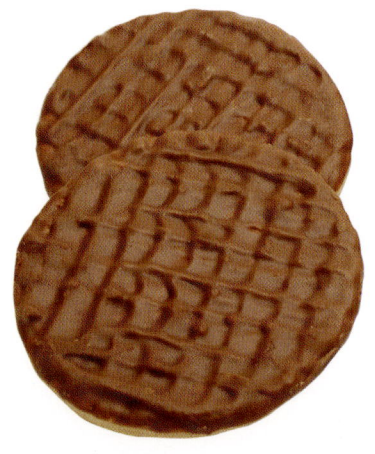

2 choc coated (single side) cookies / biscuits, 0.8 oz / 25 g

occasional snacks
cakes & desserts

The higher the fat content of the food, the smaller the serve most desserts can be. Compare your favourites with the items shown to provide a portion guide. Desserts are best kept until supper for ideal Calorie spacing.

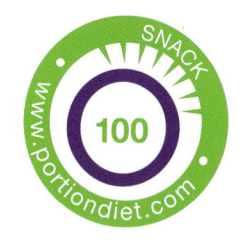

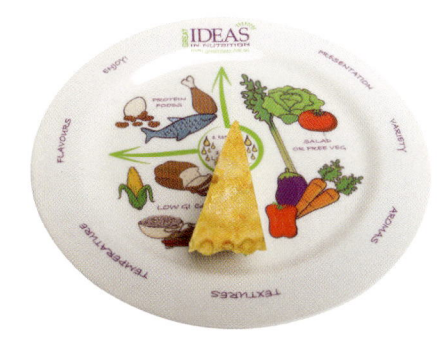

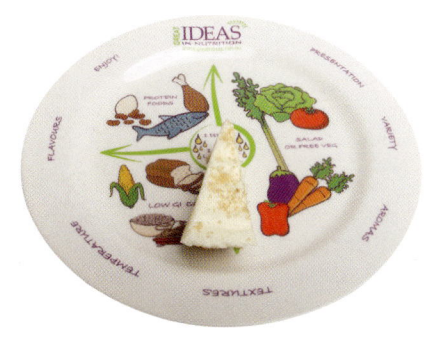

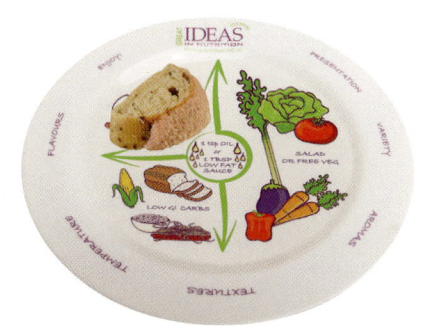

Apple pie, 1 x 1.2 in / 3 cm wedge

Cheesecake, 1 x 1.2 in / 3 cm wedge

Tea cake, unbuttered, 1 small slice

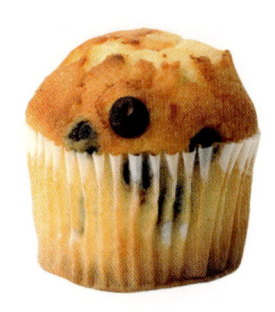

Mini muffin, 0.7 oz / 20 g

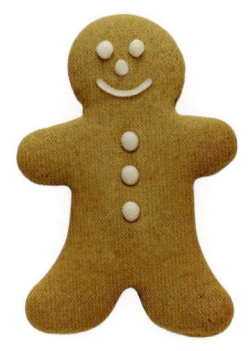

Gingerbread man, small, 1.2 oz / 35 g

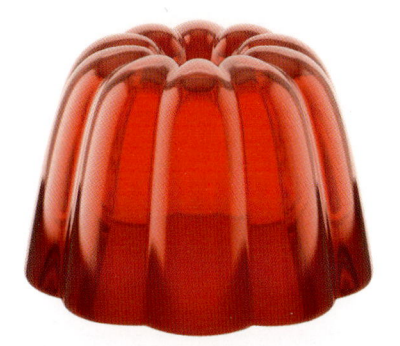

Jelly, with sugar, ¾ cup

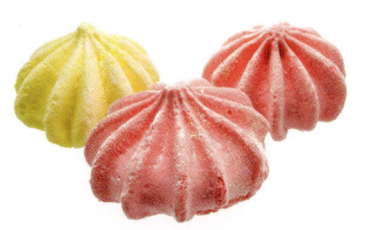

Mini meringues, 3

SNACKS | 81

occasional snacks

chocolates & lollies

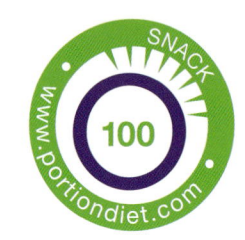

Never fall into the trap of using food as a reward for yourself or others. When you feel you need a "reward", do something nice for yourself, like giving yourself permission to spend time on yourself, reading, relaxing, playing music, fishing, pampering, or whatever suits you. These things you will look back on and be pleased you gave to yourself. "Rewarding" yourself with excess food is actually not doing something nice for yourself at all. You are likely to look back on it with regret. So choose a reward that feels good – you deserve it!

Lollies tend to be very high GI, whether the ingredients are natural or not. Those prone to diabetes would be better choosing chocolate than lollies.

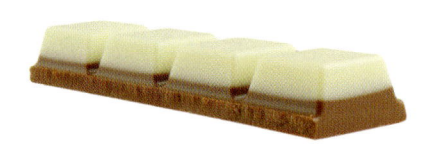

Chocolate, most brands, dark, milk or white, approx 1 x 0.7 oz / 20 g row

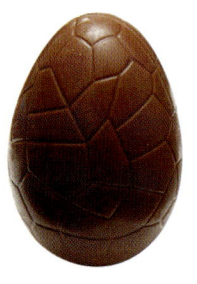

Chocolate egg, real egg sized, 0.7 oz / 20 g

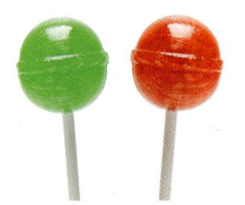

Lollipops, small, 2 x 1 oz / 30 g

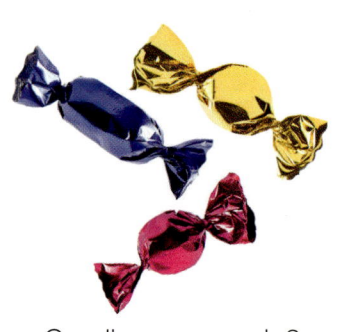

Candies, wrapped, 3

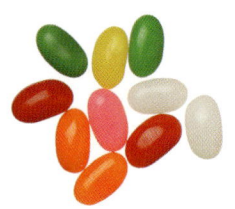

Jellybeans, 10

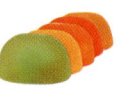

Gummy Candies / Jubes, 5

TIP If you've been a big chocolate eater in the past, you can scale down your desire by taking it out of your diet for a while. If you choose to put it back, do so in manageable quantities. Some people describe themselves as chocoholics and it is true that chocolate does have a physiological effect on sensitive people. Decide for yourself whether it can appear in your life in a healthy, occasional way.

Children learn what is normal from friends and family.

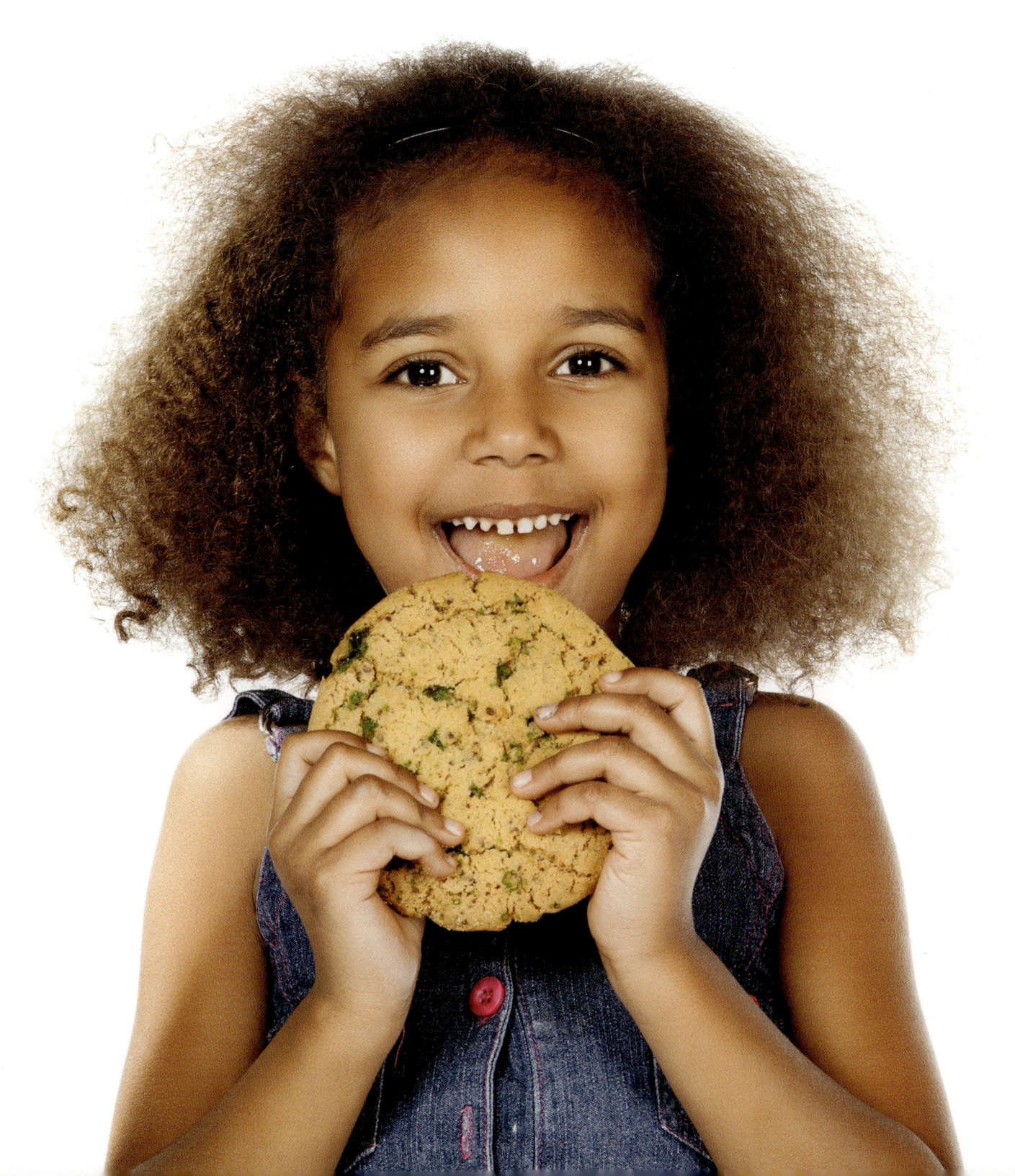

occasional snacks

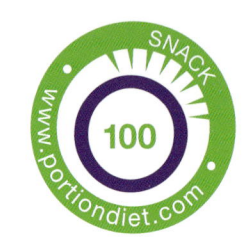

bars

Bars come in all shapes and sizes. Remember to firstly check that it has approx 100 Cals / 420 kJ (60-130 Cals / 252-546 kJ) Then check against the criteria for an everyday snack on page 74. If three out of the four criteria are not met, then the bar belongs here as an occasional choice.

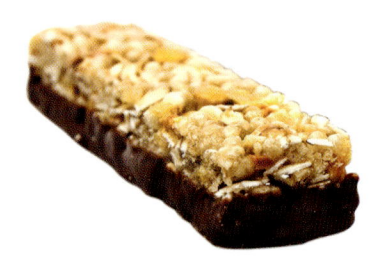

choc dipped granola / muesli bars, small, 0.7-1 oz / 20-30 g

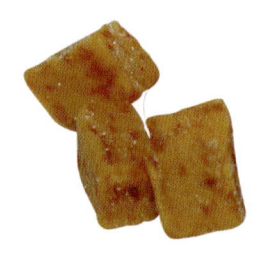

Apricot blocks, 3 x 0.3 oz / 10 g

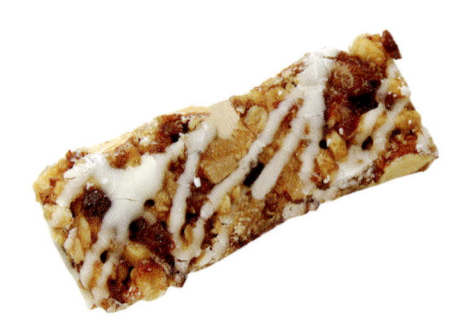

Yoghurt or chocolate drizzled bars, small, 10.7-1 oz / 20-30 g

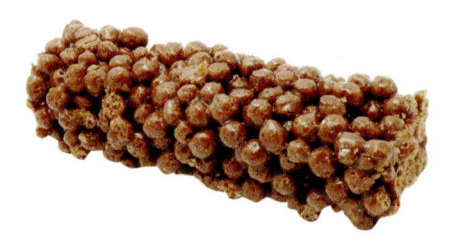

Puffed bars or those held together with syrup, 0.7-1 oz / 20-30 g

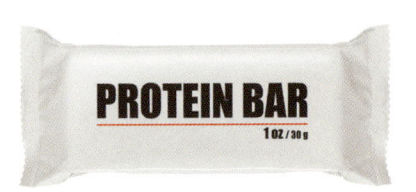

Most protein bars, 1 oz / 30 g

occasional snacks
miscellaneous

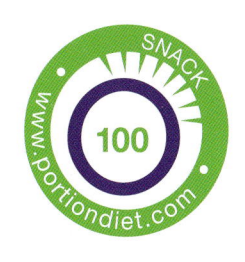

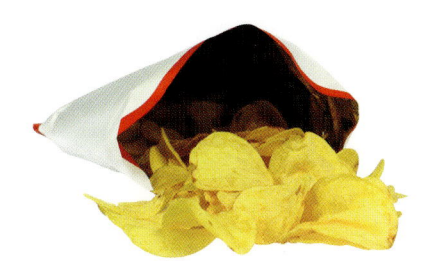

Potato crisps, all flavours, 1 x 0.7 oz / 20 g mini pack

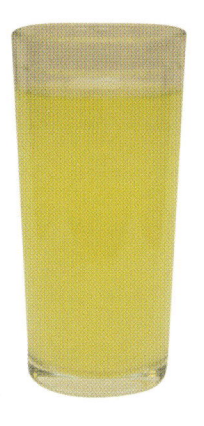

Soft drink, 6.7 fl oz / 200 ml

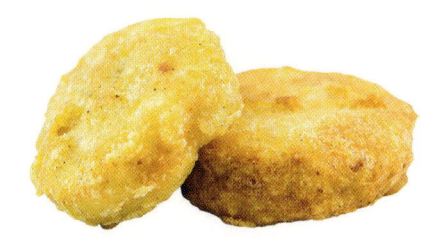

Chicken nuggets, 2 x 0.7 oz / 20 g

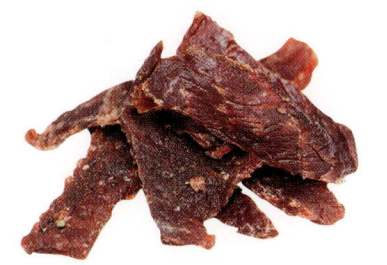

Beef jerky, 1 oz / 30 g

occasional snacks

alcohol

Alcohol has some health benefits that come along with it, but for some one glass means more. Judge for yourself whether alcohol is a problem in your life and choose healthier options for yourself.

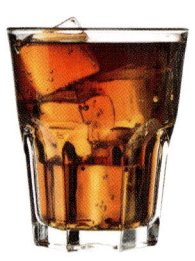

Spirit and diet mixer, most varieties, 1.5 fl oz / 45 ml spirit + 5 fl oz / 150 ml mixer

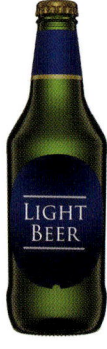

Light beer, 1 x 12 fl oz / 375 ml bottle

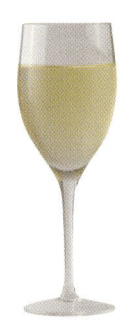

White wine, 5 fl oz / 150 ml

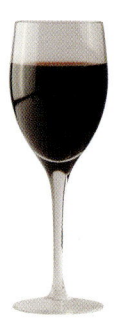

Red wine, 5 fl oz / 150 ml

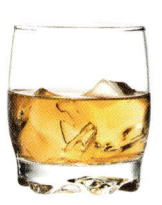

Spirits, most varieties, 1.5 fl oz / 45 ml

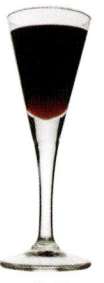

Liqueur, most varieties, 2 fl oz / 60 ml

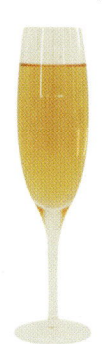

Sparkling wine, 5 fl oz / 150 ml

"200 calories is the correct amount for a weight management snack for most men, women and children. The following pages show 200 calorie serves, or you may also choose two serves from the 100 calorie section."

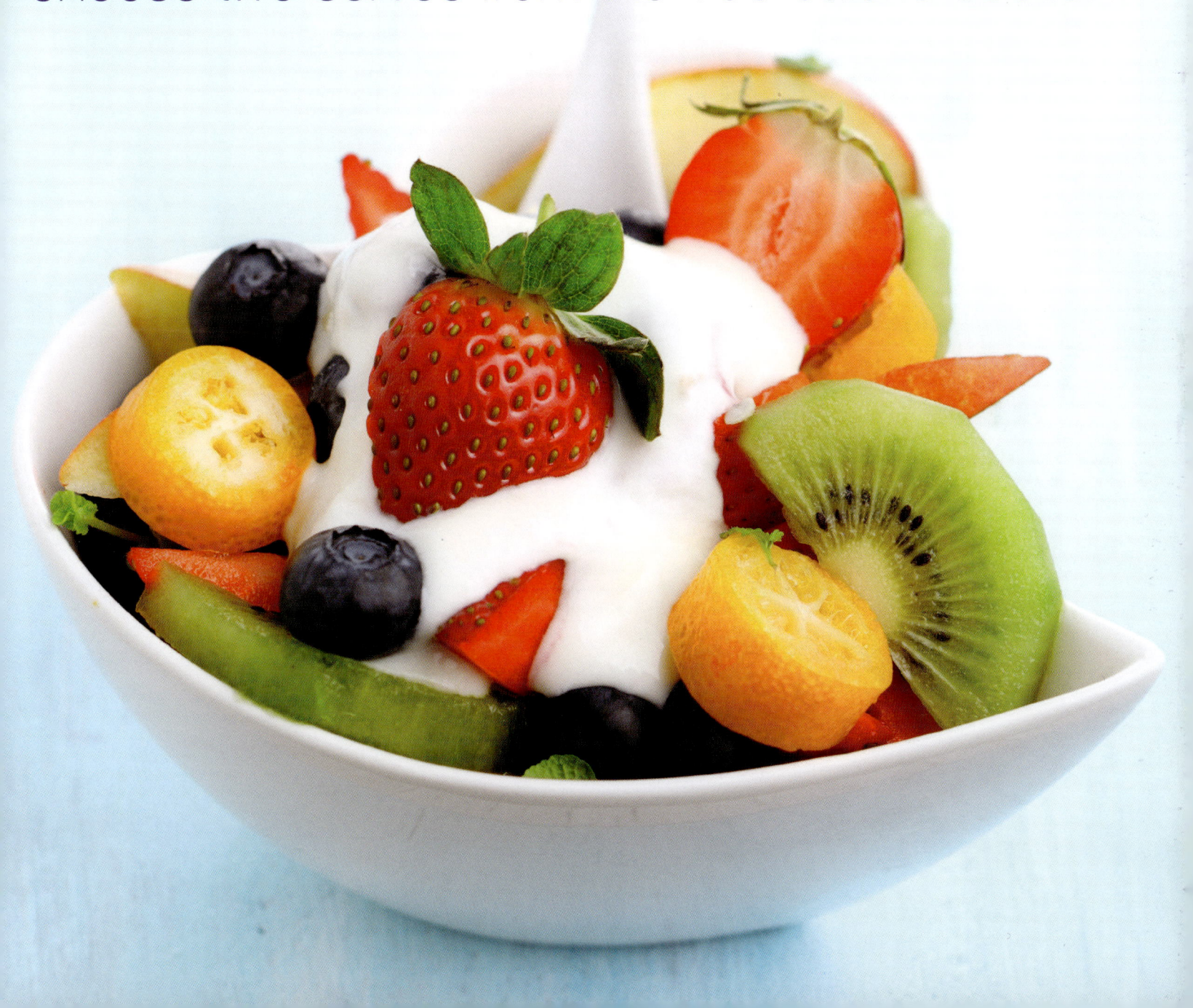

everyday snacks
dairy (e200)

Also consider 2 x e100 snacks.

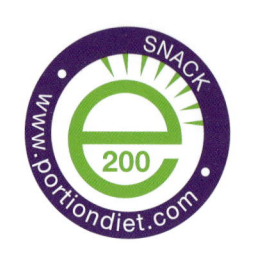

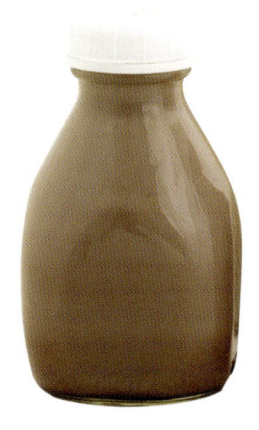

Flavoured milk, all flavours, small bottle 8.3 fl oz / 250 ml

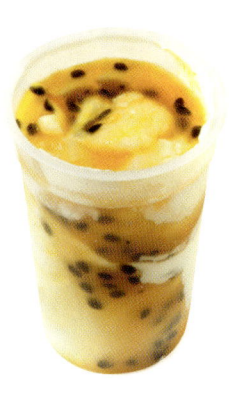

Greek yoghurt and fruit, 6.7 fl oz / 200 ml

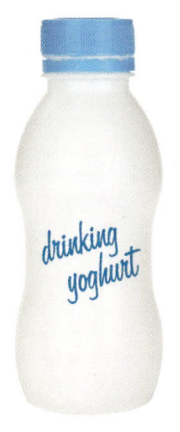

Drinking yoghurt, 6.7 fl oz / 200 ml

everyday snacks
miscellaneous (e200)

Also consider 2 x e100 snacks

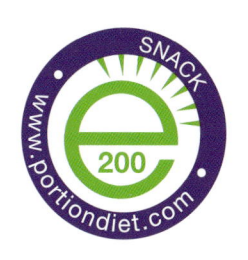

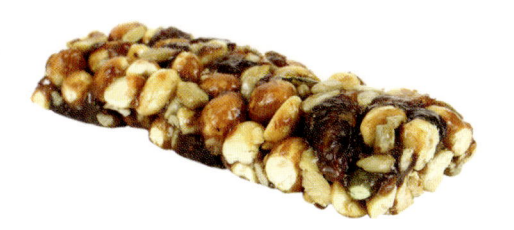

Nut bar, 1 oz / 30 g

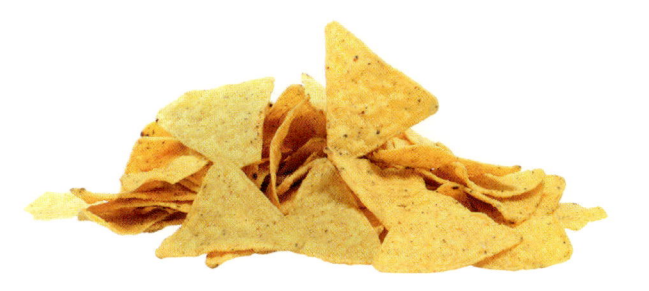

Corn or grain crisps, 1.3 oz / 40 g

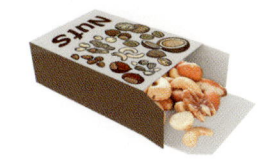

Nut snack box, 1-1.3 oz / 30-40 g

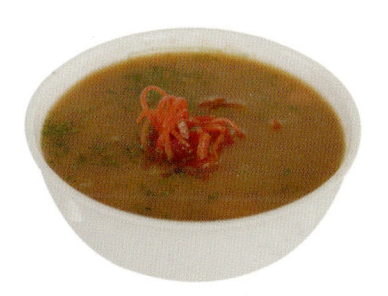

1½ cups of chunky or starchy soup

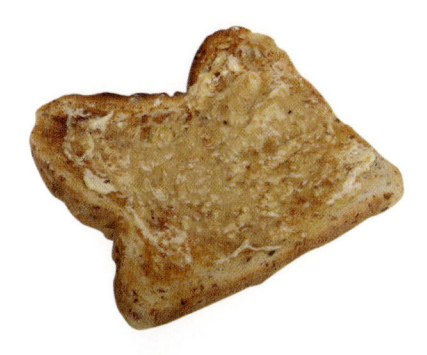

1 slice wholegrain toast with 1.5 tsp spread and 1.5 tsp peanut butter

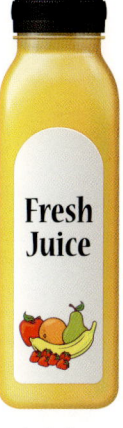

Commercial fresh juice, small-medium, 11.7 fl oz / 350 ml

SNACKS | 89

occasional snacks

o200 snacks

Also consider 2 x e/o100 snacks.

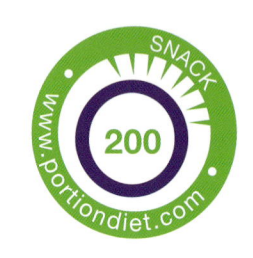

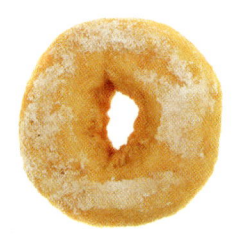

Cinnamon donut, 1 x 50 g donut

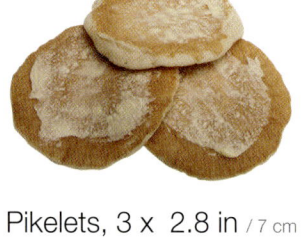

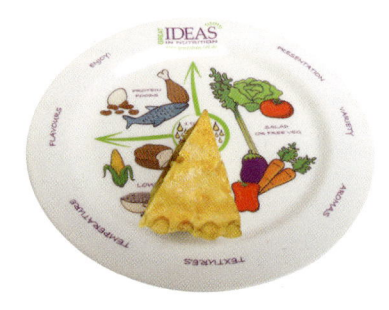

Pikelets, 3 x 2.8 in / 7 cm

Apple pie, 1 x 2.4 in / 6 cm

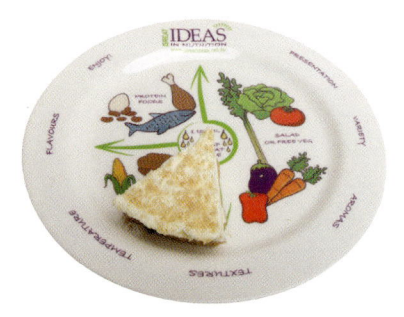

Cheesecake 1 x 2.4 in / 6 cm

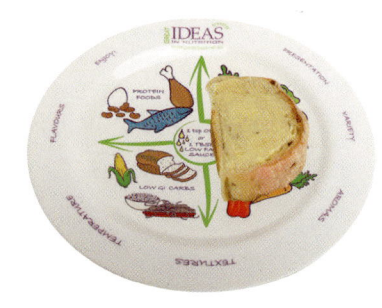

Tea cake / Boston bun, with average spread, 1 x 5 in / 13 cm wide slice

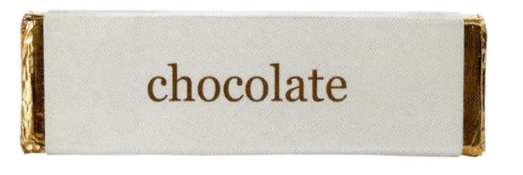

Chocolate bar, most styles 1.3 oz / 40 g

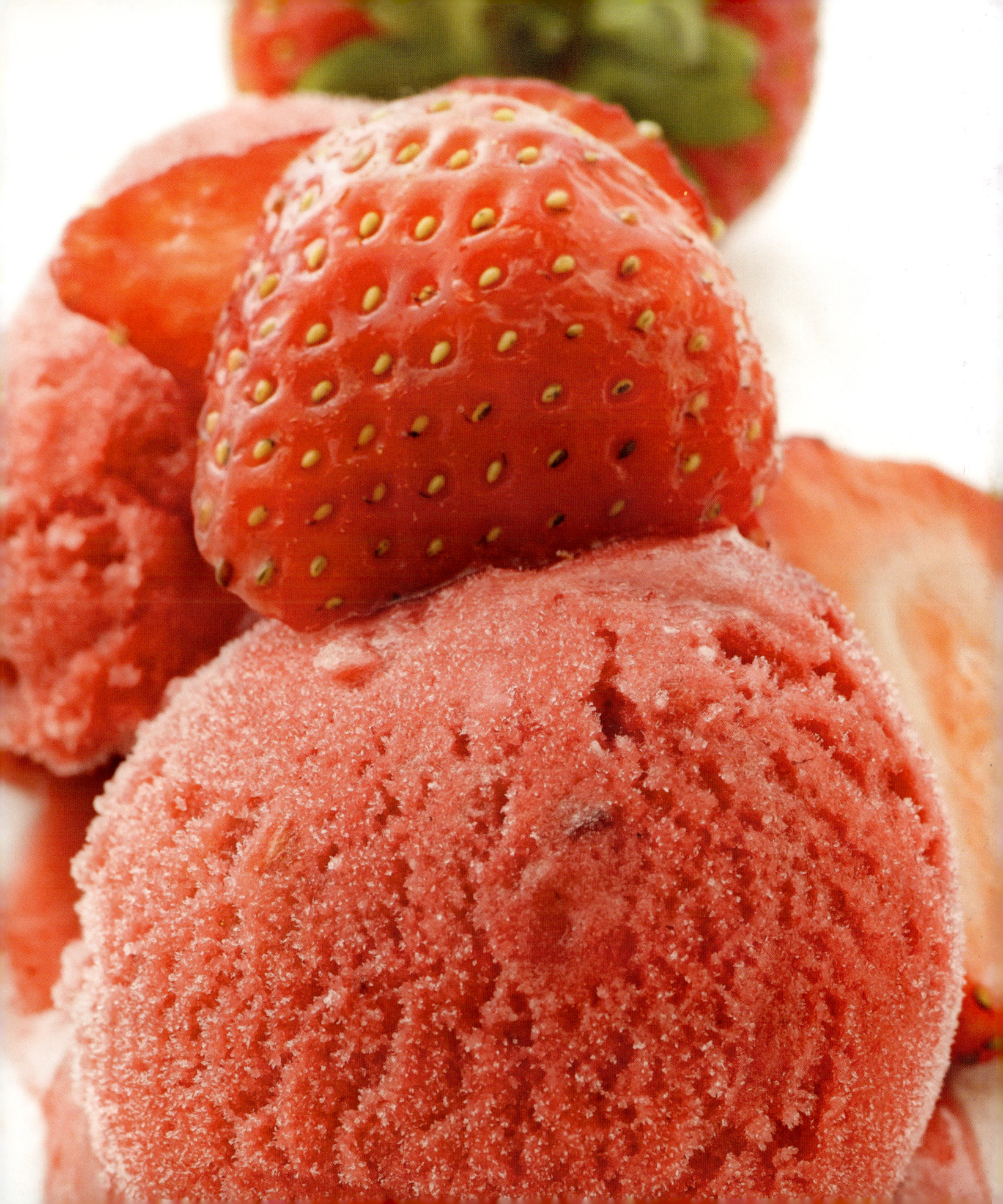

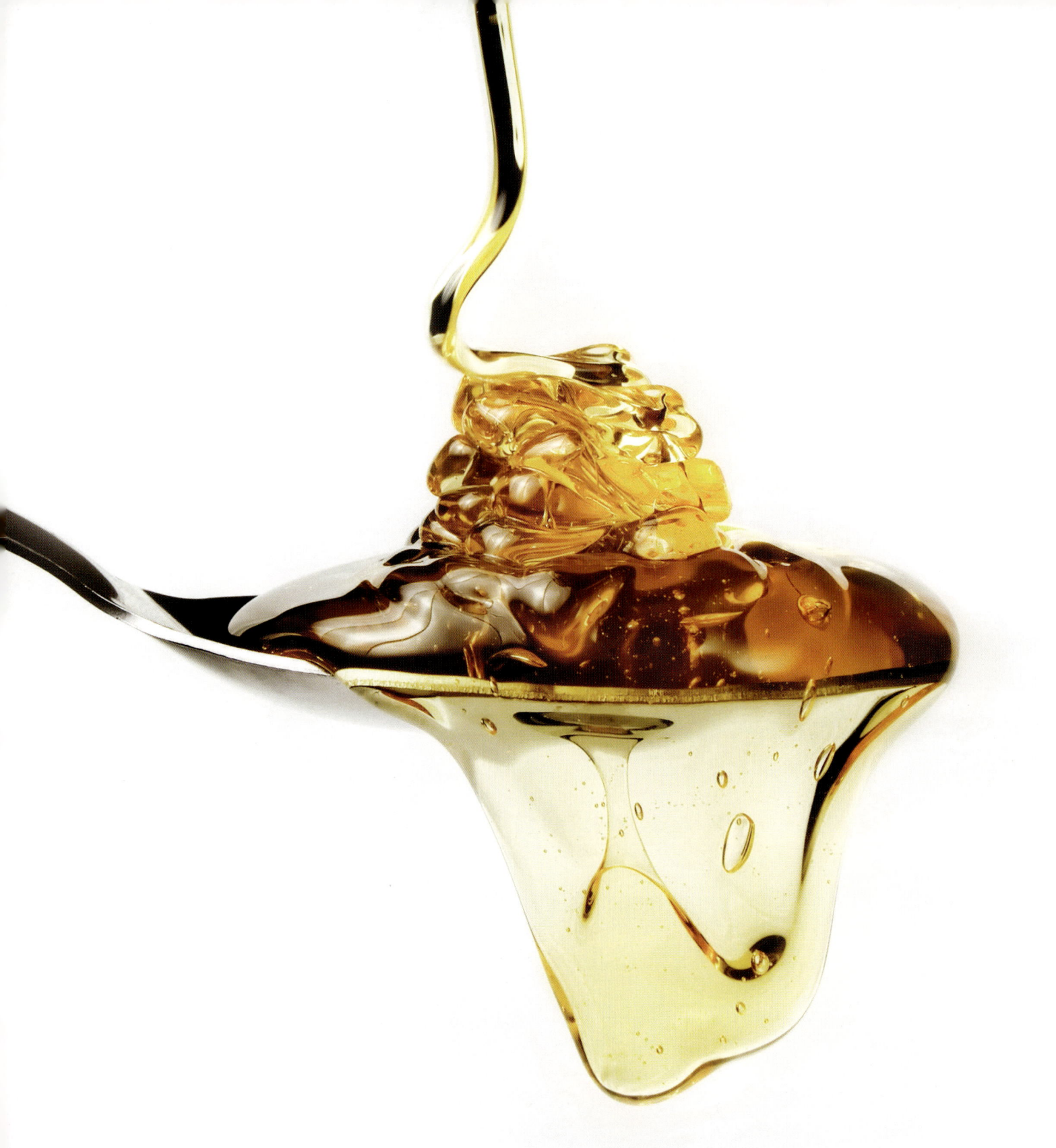

"…the larger the spoon the more we eat…"

CHAPTER 8

lunch

Lunch is often taken on the run or skipped altogether. What you choose for lunch can influence those mid-afternoon munchies. So you want to get it right most of the time.

Whether you're preparing food at home or dining out, the marker of a good choice is the vegetable content. If your usual choice consists only of bread or potato and meat it'll weigh you down for the afternoon. Choose combinations of wholegrains, protein foods and salad or vegetables.

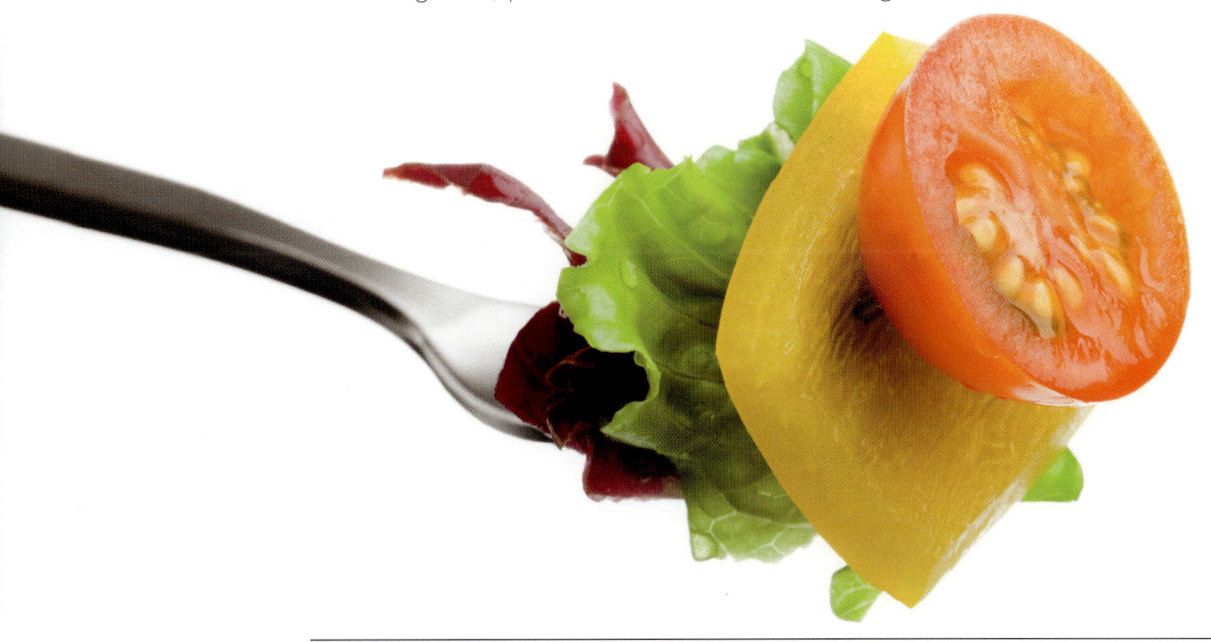

everyday menu

Sandwiches or rolls	94
Soup	98
Salads	99
Sushi	100
Kebabs	101

occasional menu

Burgers	103
Nuggets & chips	104
Fish & chips	105
Hot dog	106
Meat pie / sausage roll	107

Add your own favourites by calculating the appropriate serve from Allan Borushek's *The CalorieKing Calorie Fat and Carbohydrate Counter* or apps CalorieKing or My Fitness Pal.

everyday lunch

sandwiches or rolls

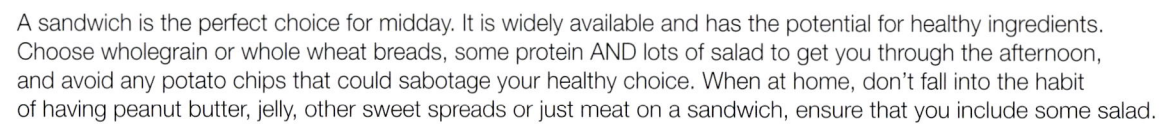

A sandwich is the perfect choice for midday. It is widely available and has the potential for healthy ingredients. Choose wholegrain or whole wheat breads, some protein AND lots of salad to get you through the afternoon, and avoid any potato chips that could sabotage your healthy choice. When at home, don't fall into the habit of having peanut butter, jelly, other sweet spreads or just meat on a sandwich, ensure that you include some salad.

Everyday breads (200 Cals / 840 kJ)

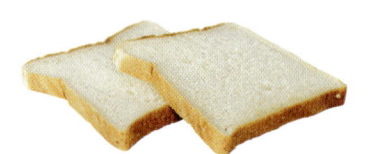

Fibre enriched white bread, 2 x 1 oz / 30 g slices

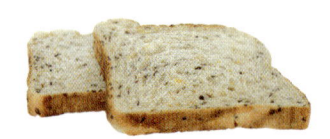

Wholegrain or seed bread, 2 x 1 oz / 30 g slices

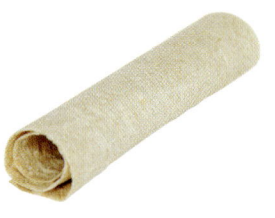

Flat bread, 1.9 oz / 56 g

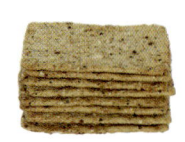

Wholegrain crackers, 8

Pocket bread, 2.2 oz / 65 g

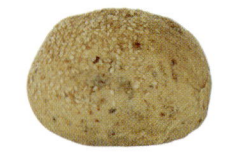

Grain roll, small, 2 oz / 60 g

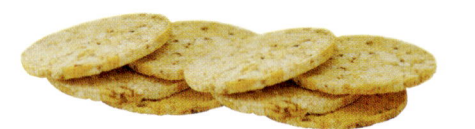

Grainy rice / corn cakes, 8 thin or 6 thick, 1.8 oz / 55 g

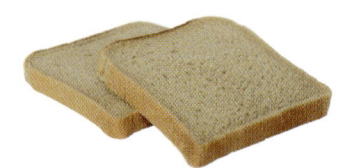

Rye bread, 2 x 1 oz / 30 g slices

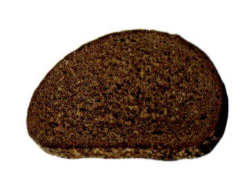

Dark rye bread, 1 slice, 2.3 oz / 70 g

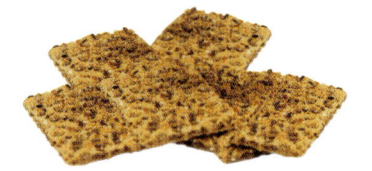

Wholegrain crispbread, 5 pieces

Occasional breads (200 Cals / 840 kJ)

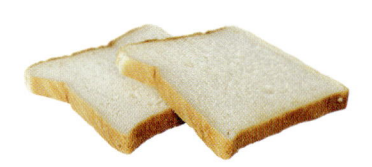

Bread, white, 2 x 1 oz / 30 g slices

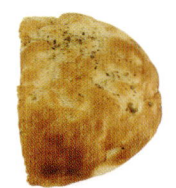

Foccacia, ²⁄₃ roll, 2.7 oz / 50 g

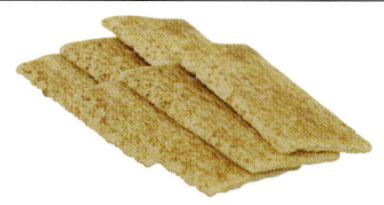

Puffed crispbread, 1.2 oz / 35 g

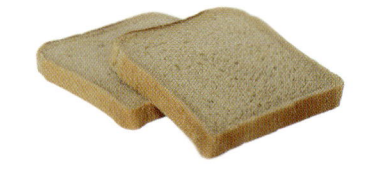

Whole wheat bread, 2 x 1 oz / 30 g slices

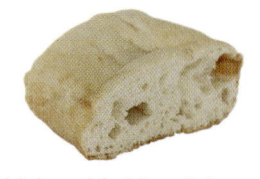

Turkish bread / white roll, 2 oz / 60 g

Example: Melissa, on 350 Cals / 1470 kJ, could choose to make a sandwich with two slices of multigrain bread, fill it with 1oz / 30 g chicken, spread it with 2 tsp of fat free mayonnaise and ¹⁄₃ of an avocado, and then load it with lettuce, tomato, mushrooms and sprouts.

everyday lunch

sandwiches continued

Meal components

Cals / kJ	Bread (200 Cals / 840 kJ)	Protein (50 Cals / 210 kJ)	Add Ons (100 Cals / 420 kJ)	Free Foods
350 / 1470 ✓	1 serve	1	1	1
450 / 1890 ✓✓	1 serve	2	1.5	1
550 / 2310 ✓	1 serve	4	1.5	2

Protein (50 Cals / 210 kJ)

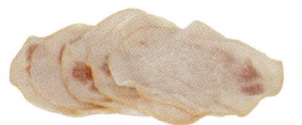

Ham, 1.3 oz / 40 g

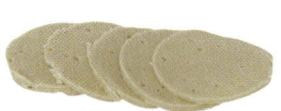

Vegetarian deli meat, 1 oz / 30 g

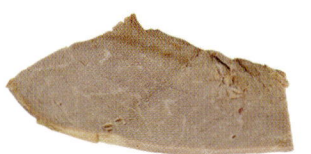

Roast or corned beef, 1.3 oz / 40 g

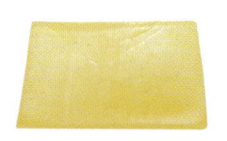

Cheese, min 50% less fat, 0.7 oz / 20 g

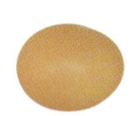

1 egg, small, boiled

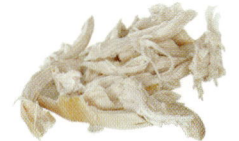

Chicken, 1 oz / 30 g

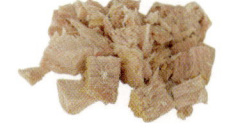

Tuna or salmon, 1.3 oz / 40 g

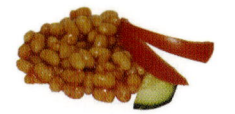

Baked beans, 2.2 oz / 65 g

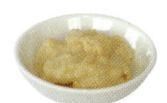

Hommous, 1.3 oz / 16 g

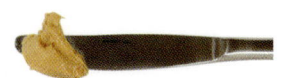

Peanut butter, 1.5 tsp

Some 'Add On' ideas (100 Cals / 420 kJ)

*For more 'Add Ons' serves refer to Appendix 2

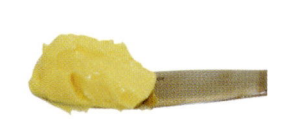

Butter or margarine, 3 tsp

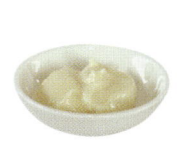

Mayonnaise, 3 tsp

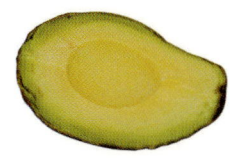

Avocado, 1/3, 2 oz / 60 g

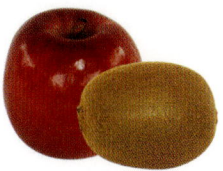

Fruit, small, 2 pieces

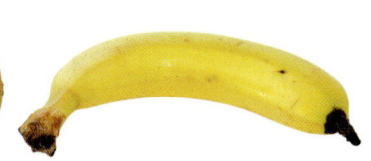

1 large piece of fruit

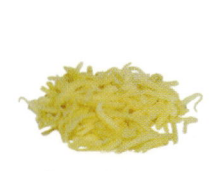

Grated cheese, 0.7 oz / 20 g

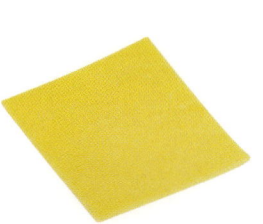

Cheese, full fat, 0.7 oz / 20 g

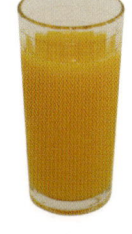

Juice, 6.7 fl oz / 200 ml

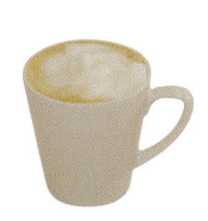

Cappucino, skim, 8.3-11.7 fl oz / 250-350 ml

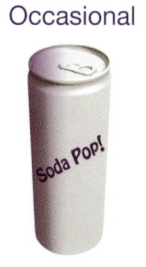

Occasional

Soda / softdrink, small can, 7.5 fl oz / 225 ml

Continued over ▶

LUNCH | 95

everyday lunch

sandwiches continued

Add up to a cupful of salad plus one other free food such as pickles or parmesan.

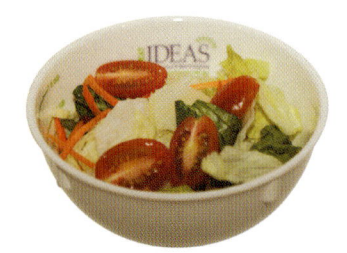

1 cup salad

Some 'Free Food' ideas (<20 Cals / 85 kJ) *For more 'Free Foods' serves refer to Appendix 3

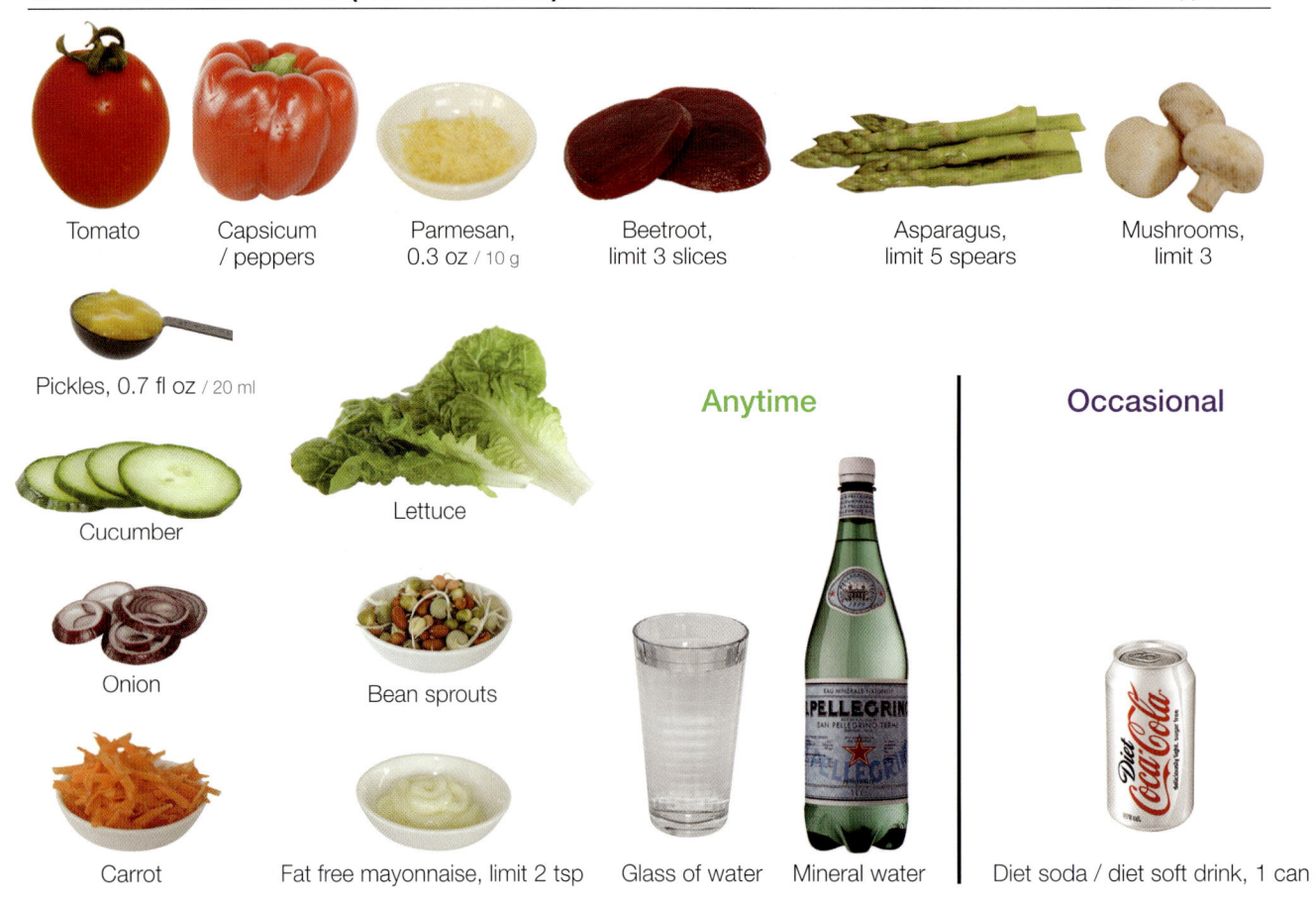

- Tomato
- Capsicum / peppers
- Parmesan, 0.3 oz / 10 g
- Beetroot, limit 3 slices
- Asparagus, limit 5 spears
- Mushrooms, limit 3
- Pickles, 0.7 fl oz / 20 ml
- Cucumber
- Lettuce
- Onion
- Bean sprouts
- Carrot
- Fat free mayonnaise, limit 2 tsp

Anytime
- Glass of water
- Mineral water

Occasional
- Diet soda / diet soft drink, 1 can

"A sandwich is the perfect choice for midday."

"The colours of vegetables reflect their nutritional properties. Eat a rainbow daily."

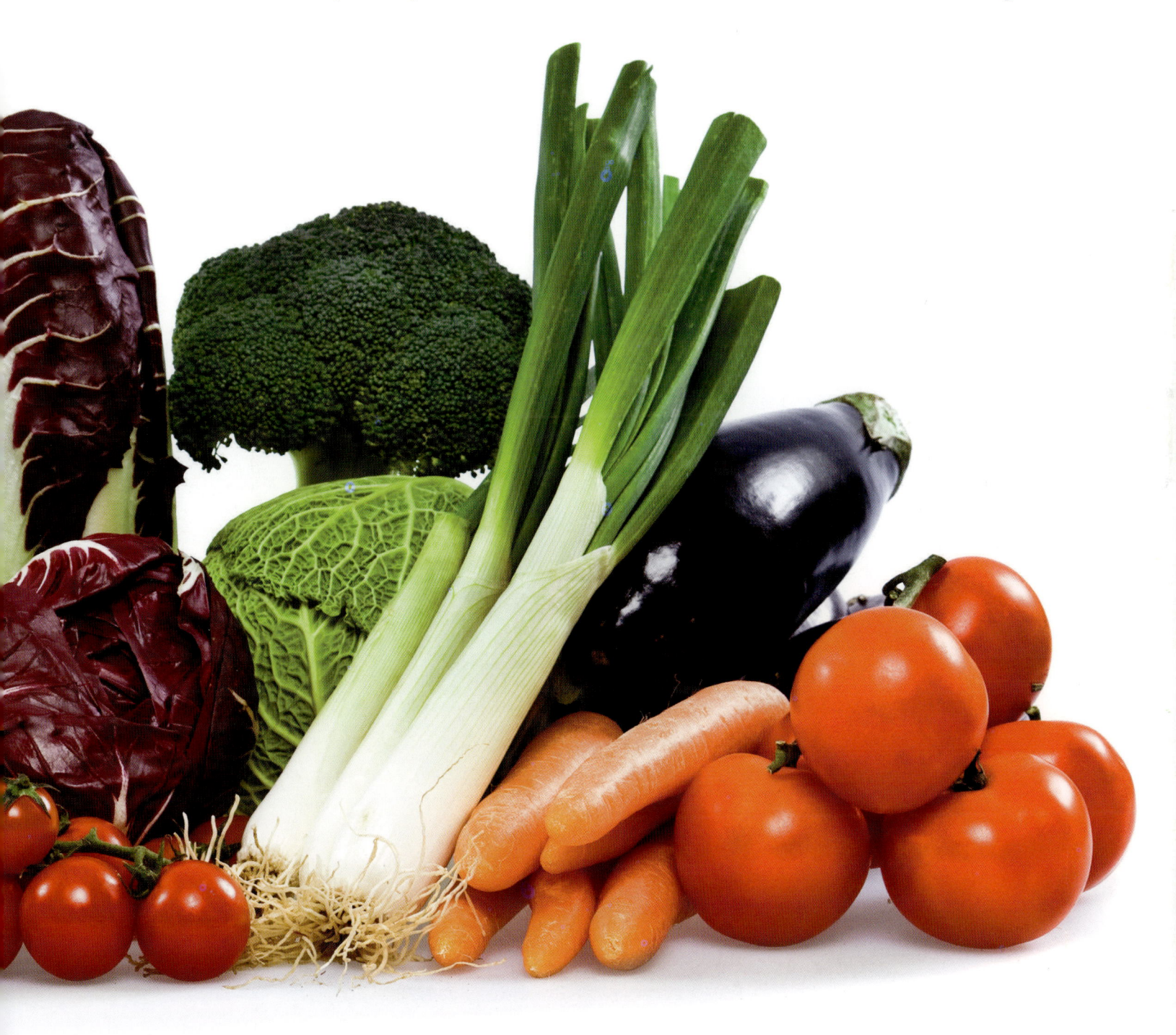

everyday lunch

soup

Most canned or home made soups, e.g., lamb and vegetable, minestrone, chicken and corn, sweet potato. Choose low-salt canned soups. Avoid soups with added oil or cream.

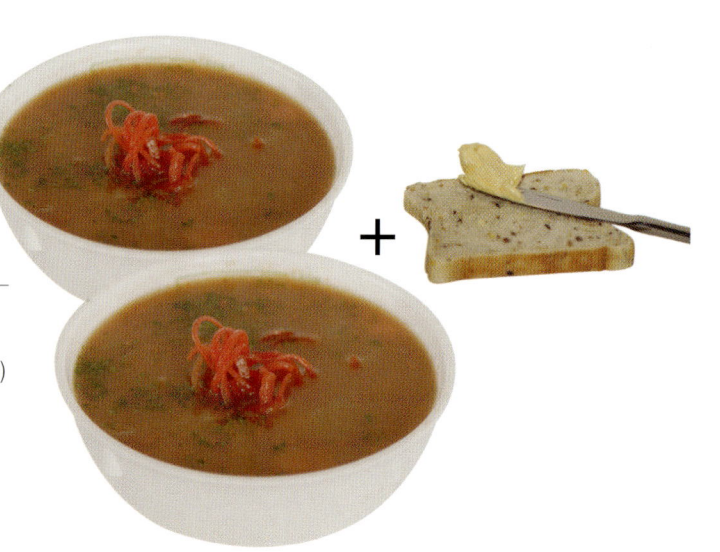

350 Calories / 1470 kJ

1½ cups starchy/chunky soup (200 Cals / 840 kJ)
+ 1 bread serve (100 Cals / 420 kJ)
+ 1½ tsp butter or margarine (50 Cals / 210 kJ)

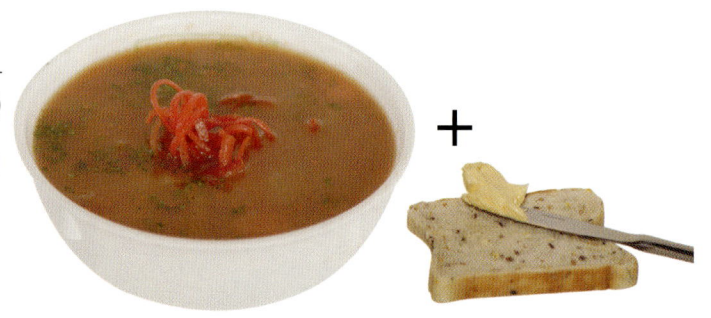

450 Calories / 1890 kJ

1½ cups soup (200 Cals / 840 kJ)
+ 2 bread serves (200 Cals / 840 kJ)
+ 1½ tsp butter or margarine (50 Cals / 210 kJ)

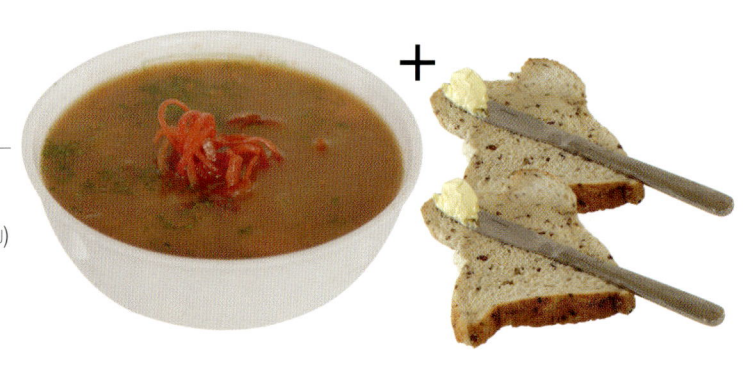

550 Calories / 2310 kJ

2 bowls soup (3 cups) (400 Cals / 1680 kJ)
+ 1 bread serve (100 Cals / 420 kJ)
+ 1½ tsp butter or margarine (50 Cals / 210 kJ)

98 | LUNCH

everyday lunch

salads

A great alternative to sandwiches, salads on a plate might take a bit more planning, but they're worth it. Try a pre-packed green salad for a quick source of greens.

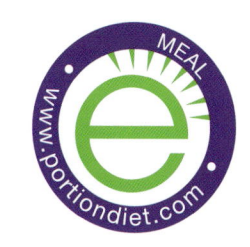

350 Calories / 1470 kJ

3 protein serves (see page 95) (150 Cals / 630 kJ)
+ ¾ cup starchy salad (150 Cals / 630 kJ)
+ 1½ cups free salads (30 Cals / 125 kJ)
+ 1 Free Food, (e.g., dressing) (20 Cals / 85 kJ)

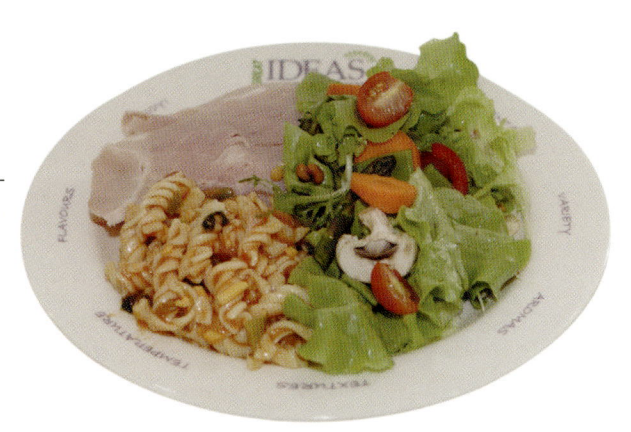

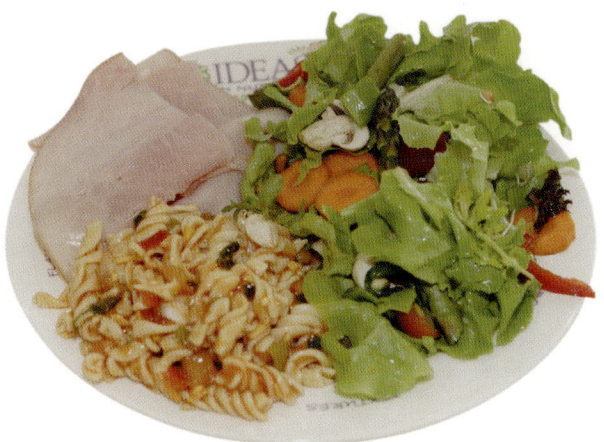

450 Calories / 1890 kJ

4 protein serves (200 Cals / 840 kJ) (see page 95)
+ 1 cup starchy salad (200 Cals / 840 kJ)
+ 2 cups free salad (30 Cals / 125 kJ)
+ 1 Free Food, (e.g., dressing) (20 Cals / 85 kJ)

550 Calories / 2310 kJ

4 protein serves (see page 95) (200 Cals / 840 kJ)
+ 1 cup starchy salad (200 Cals / 840 kJ)
+ 2 cups free salad (30 Cals / 125 kJ)
+ 1 Free Food, (e.g., dressing) (20 Cals / 85 kJ)
+ 1 Add On (e.g., avocado) (100 Cals / 420 kJ)

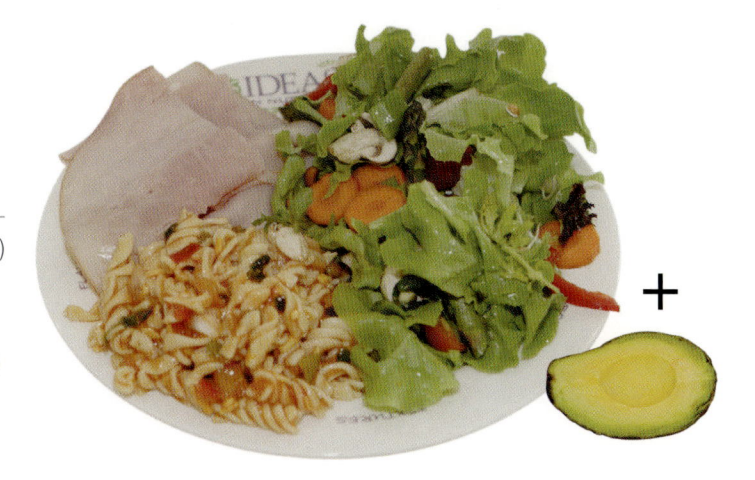

LUNCH | 99

everyday lunch

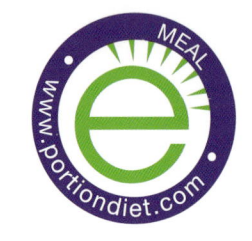

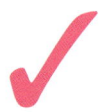

sushi

Sushi is becoming a very convenient lunch. It's nice and petite, so you only expect to eat a small volume. You don't get a lot of vegetable or protein intake from this choice, but it's still pretty healthy. Most sushi is relatively low GI.

✓ **350 Calories** / 1470 kJ
6 sushi pieces

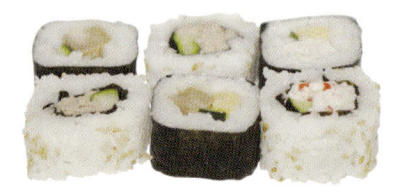

✓ **450 Calories** / 1890 kJ
8 sushi pieces

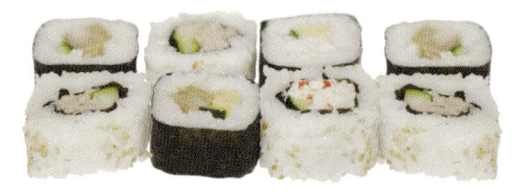

✓ **550 Calories** / 2310 kJ
10 sushi pieces

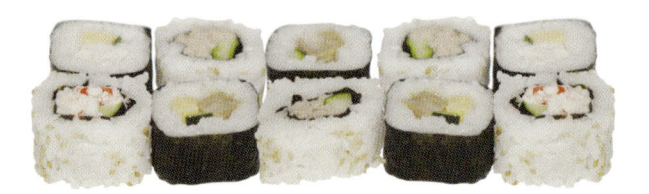

"What we eat is certainly a problem for some. How much we eat is becoming a problem for all of us."

everyday lunch

kebab

A kebab is easily available in many shopping centres, and can be a healthy choice with a bit of planning. The average doner kebab has 650 Calories / 2730 kJ, so you want to go easy on the meal deal options. Here are some ways you can make a kebab an everyday healthy choice and achieve your weight control goals.

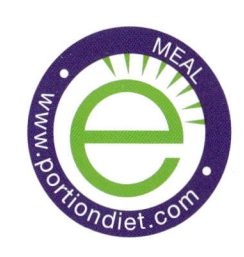

350 Calories / 1470 kJ

Felafel kebab (no cheese) or snack sized meat kebab with sweet chilli or BBQ sauce

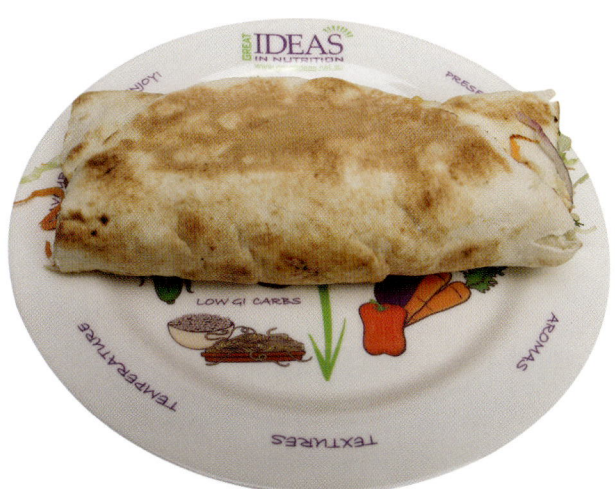

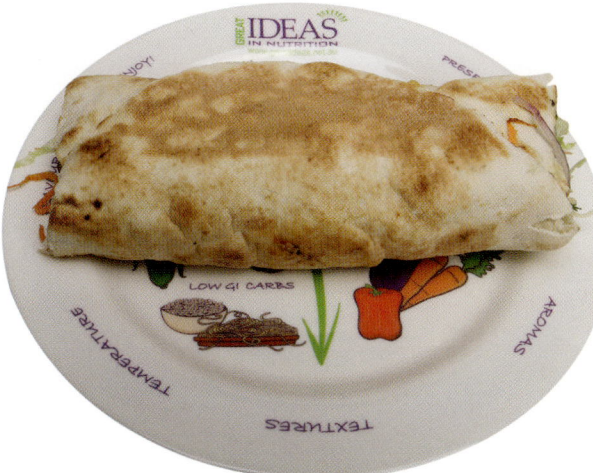

450 Calories / 1890 kJ

Standard sized meat kebab (no cheese) with sweet chilli or BBQ sauce

550 Calories / 2310 kJ

Standard sized meat kebab
+ 1 Add On (e.g., cheese, pineapple, 1/3 avocado or creamy sauce)
(100 Cals / 420 kJ)

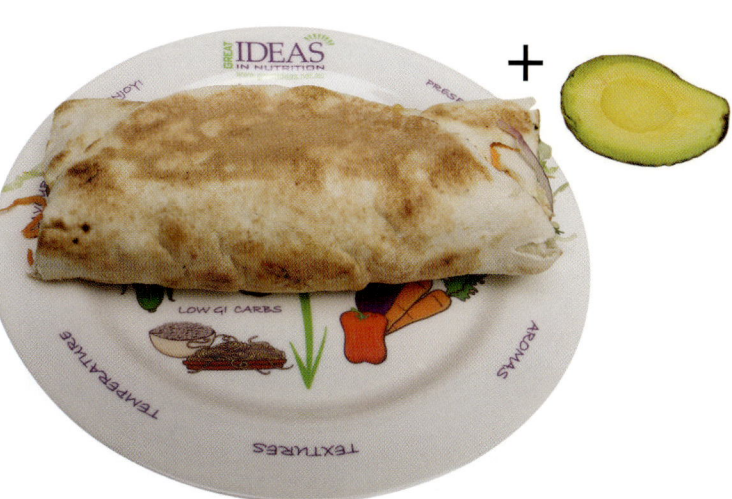

LUNCH | 101

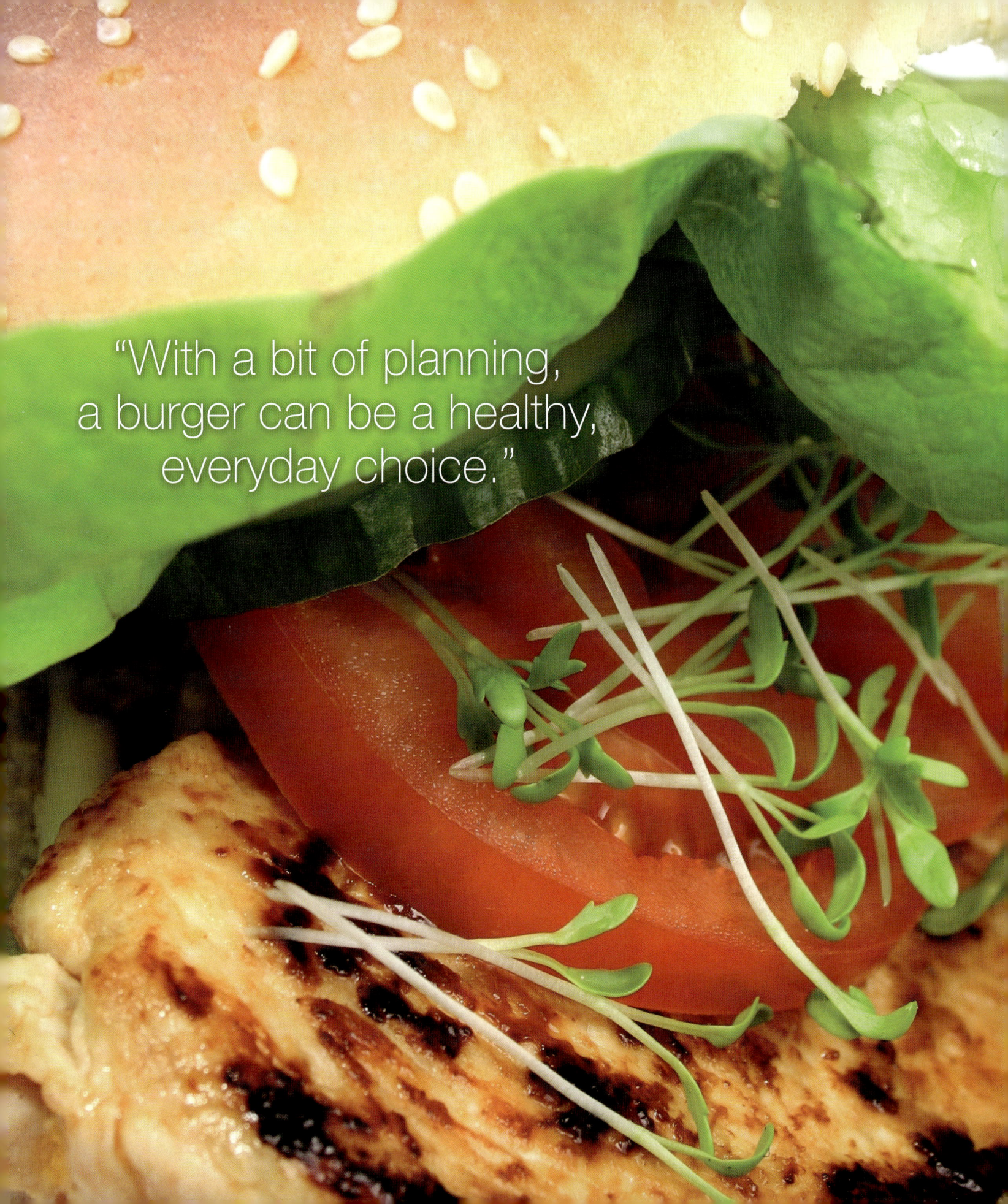

"With a bit of planning, a burger can be a healthy, everyday choice."

occasional lunch

burgers

While burgers have been categorised as an occasional choice here, it is because they usually only come on white rolls and the meat quality may be poor. With a bit of planning, a burger can be a healthy everyday choice. Removing the top half of a bun and eating on a plate is ideal when possible.

Meal components

Cals / kJ	Bun (150 Cals / 630 kJ)	Patty (200 Cals / 840 kJ)	Free Veg (<20 Cals / 85 kJ)	Add Ons (100 Cals / 420 kJ)
350 / 1470 ✓	1	1	1	0
450 / 1890 ✓✓	1	1	1	1
550 / 2310 ✓	2	1	1	½

Bun (150 Cals / 630 kJ)

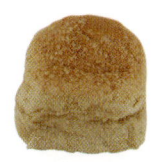

Small bread roll

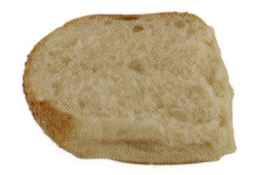

½ large hamburger bun

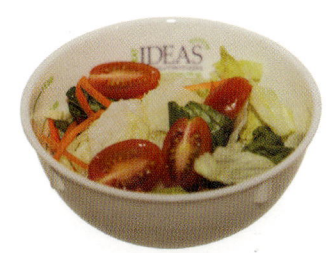

Free veg (<20 Cals / 85 kJ)

Bowl of salad or any salad ingredients

Beef, vege, chicken or fish patty (200 Cals / 840 kJ)

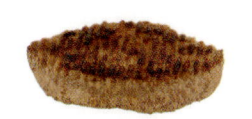

Beef patty

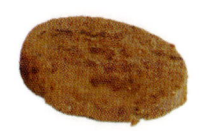

Vege patty

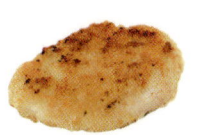

Chicken patty

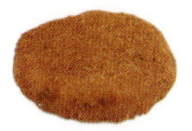

Fish patty

Add Ons (100 Cals / 420 kJ)

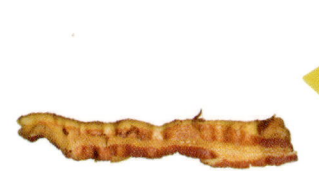

Bacon, 1 regular or 2 Canadian / centre cut slices

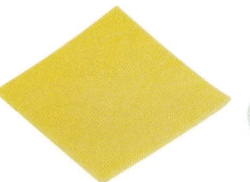

Cheese, 1 slice, 1 oz / 30 g

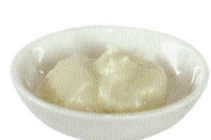

Mayonnaise, 3 tsp

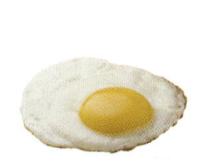

Egg, fried, 1

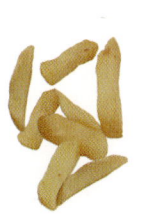

Fries, 8 thick cut or 14 thin, 1.7 oz / 50 g

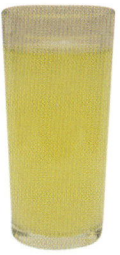

Soda / soft drink, 1 glass, 6.7 fl oz / 200 ml

LUNCH | 103

occasional lunch

nuggets & chips

You don't get much for your Calorie spend here. Try to eat slowly, leaving the fries until last so they are cooler and it is easier to stop at the right amount for you.

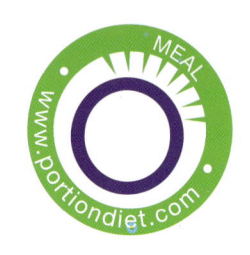

350 Calories / 1470 kJ

4 nuggets (200 Cals / 840 kJ)
+ 8 chips 1.7 oz / 50 g (150 Cals / 630 kJ)

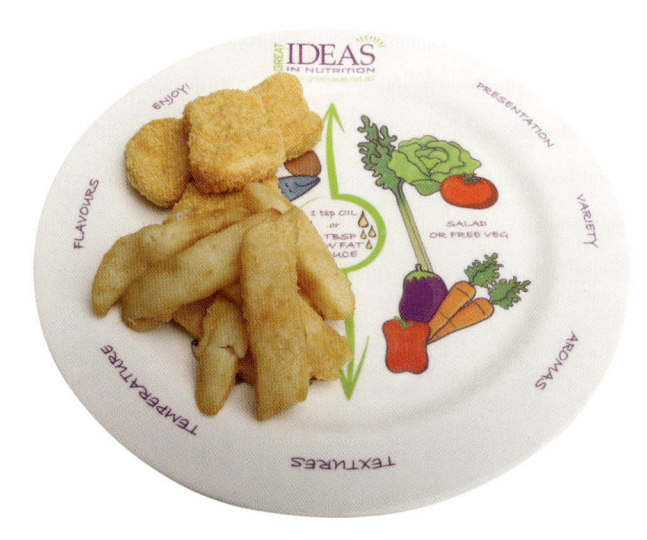

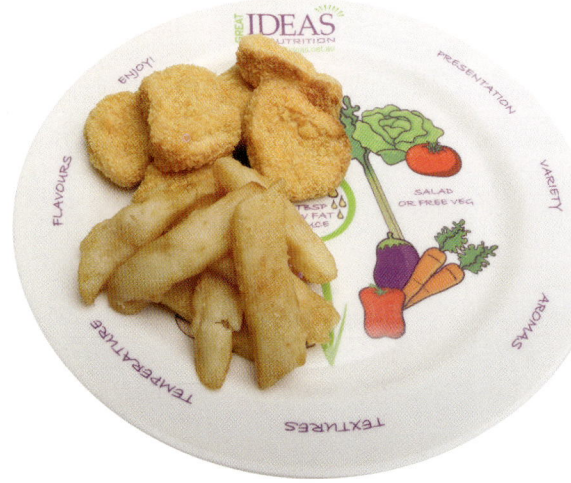

450 Calories / 1890 kJ

6 nuggets (300 Cals / 1260 kJ)
+ 8 chips 1.7 oz / 50 g (150 Cals / 630 kJ)

550 Calories / 2310 kJ

6 nuggets (300 Cals / 1260 kJ)
+ 8 chips 1.7 oz / 50 g (150 Cals / 630 kJ)
+ small can of soda / soft drink, 6.7 fl oz / 200 ml

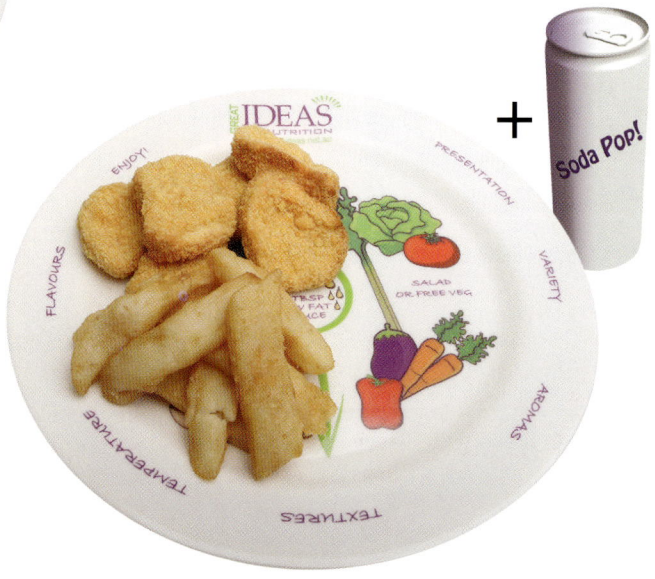

> **TIP** Natural colour is a guide to vitamin variety. Note the lack of colour variation in these options.

occasional lunch

fish & chips

This tasty fingerfood is full of fat and usually the worst kind. Cooking fish and potatoes at home in olive or canola oil can certainly improve this combination but it still lacks some colour from vegetables. If you like this option, aim to spend most of your Calories on the fish and look for outlets where you can buy salad instead of fries.

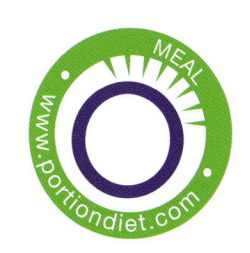

350 Calories / 1470 kJ

1 battered fish fillet, 6 inch / 16 cm long
(300 Cals / 1260 kJ)
+ 3 chips, 0.5 oz / 15 g (50 Cals / 210 kJ)

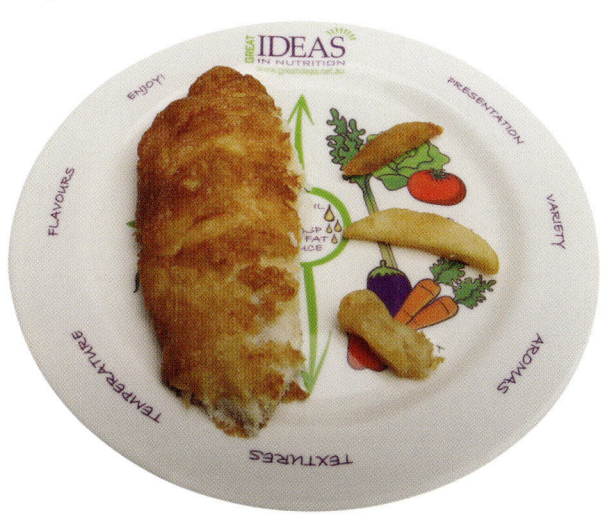

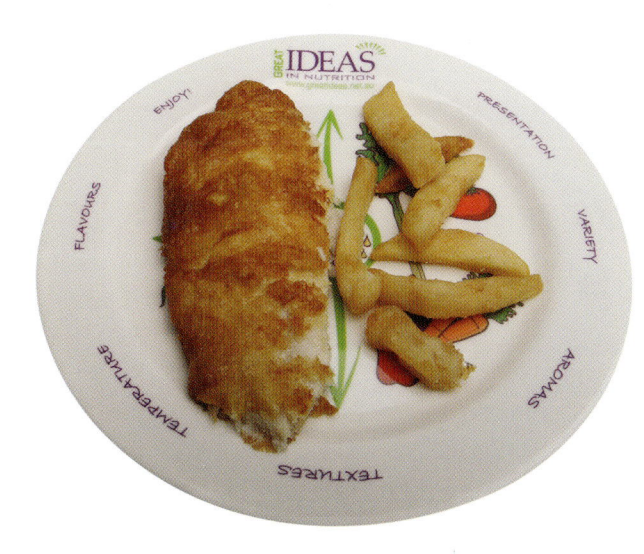

450 Calories / 1890 kJ

1 battered fish fillet, 6 inch / 16 cm long
(300 Cals / 1260 kJ)
+ 6–8 chips, 1.7 oz / 50 g (150 Cals / 630 kJ)

550 Calories / 2310 kJ

1 battered fish fillet, 6 inch / 16 cm long
(300 Cals / 1260 kJ)
+ 10–15 chips, 3 oz / 90 g (250 Cals / 1050 kJ)

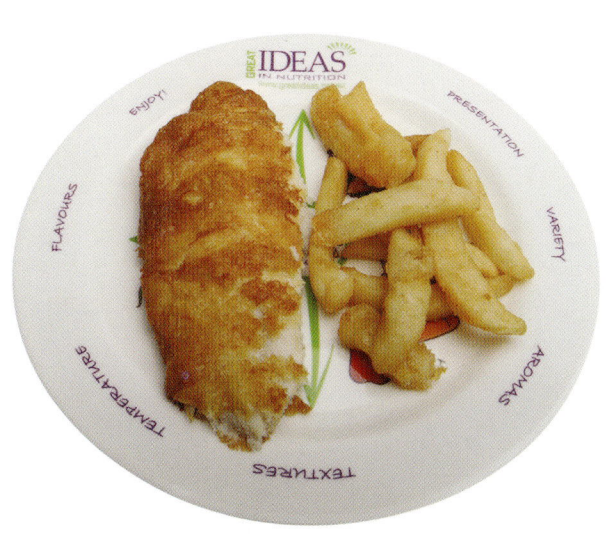

LUNCH

occasional lunch

hot dog

Don't forget to be mindful when eating this occasional sporting favourite. Ketchup, mustard or onions increase the calories only a small amount while cheese, mayonnaise and your choice of drink can make the difference between weight loss, maintenance or gain.

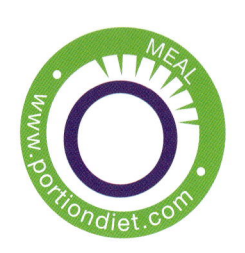

350 Calories / 1470 kJ

1 hot dog (180 Cals / 756 kJ)
+ bun (150 Cals / 630 kJ)
+ 0.7 fl oz / 20 ml ketchup / mustard (20 Cals / 84 kJ)

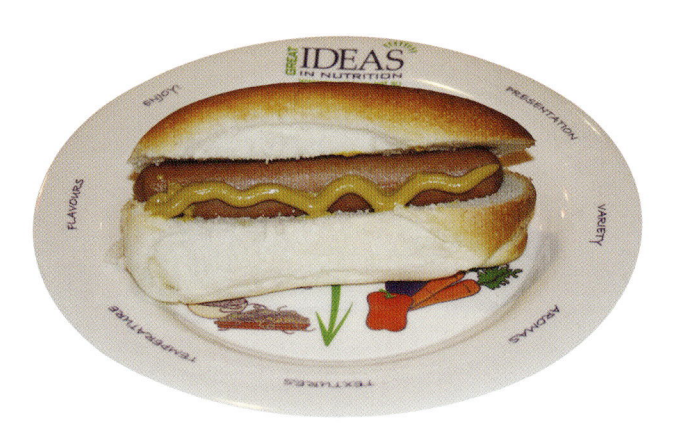

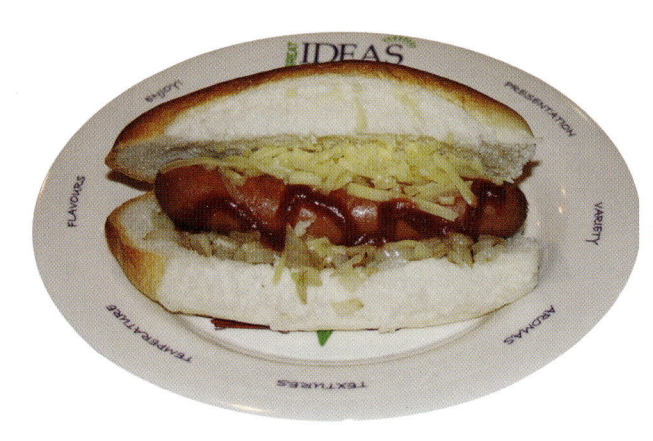

450 Calories / 1890 kJ

1 hot dog (180 Cals / 756 kJ)
+ bun (150 Cals / 630 kJ)
+ 0.7 fl oz / 20 ml ketchup / mustard (20 Cals / 84 kJ)
+ 0.5 oz / 15 g cheese (75 cals / 315 kJ)
+ ¼ cup fried onion (20 cals / 84 kJ)

550 Calories / 2310 kJ

1 hot dog (180 Cals / 756 kJ)
+ bun (150 Cals / 630 kJ)
+ 0.7 fl oz / 20 ml ketchup / mustard (20 Cals / 84 kJ)
+ 0.5 oz / 15 g cheese (75 cals / 315 kJ)
+ ¼ cup fried onion (20 cals / 84 kJ)
+ 6.7 fl oz / 200 ml soda

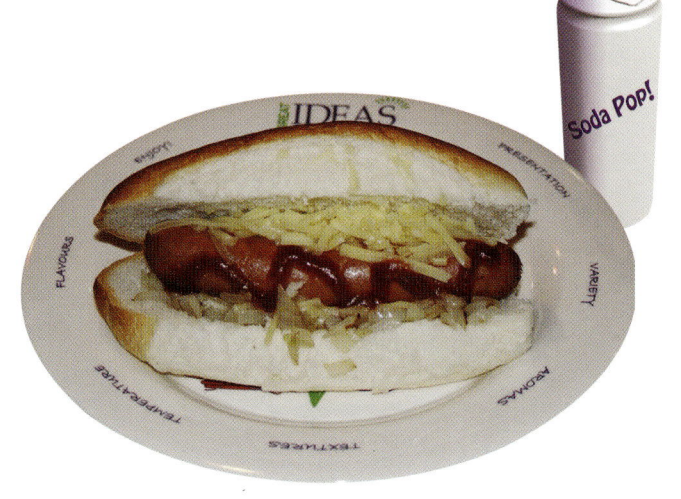

occasional lunch

meat pie/sausage roll

Meat pies and sausage rolls vary in content and size significantly. An average representation is shown here. Add an additional free serve if you like sauce.

350 Calories / 1470 kJ

Small sausage roll
+ 1 Free Food
(e.g., 0.7 fl oz / 20 ml ketchup)

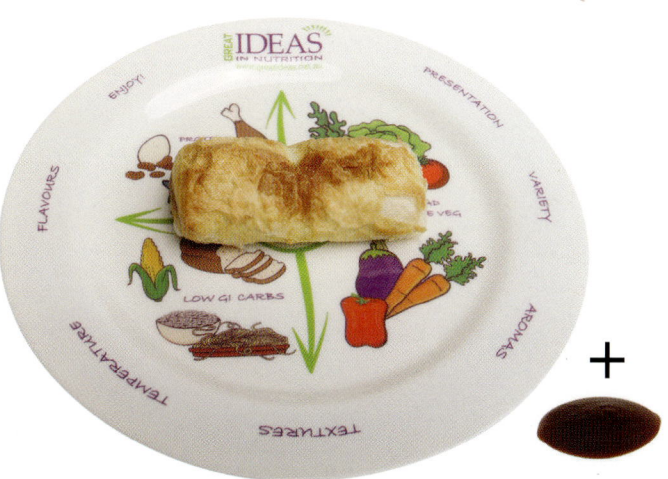

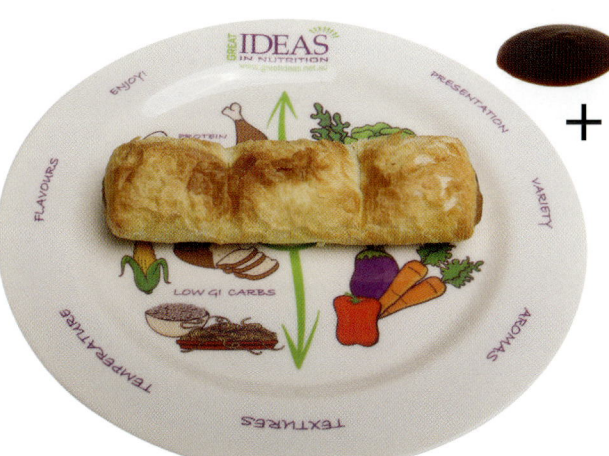

450 Calories / 1890 kJ

1 standard sausage roll
+ 1 Free Food
(e.g., 0.7 fl oz / 20 ml ketchup)

550 Calories / 2310 kJ

1 standard meat pie
+ 1 Free Food
(e.g., 0.7 fl oz / 20 ml ketchup)

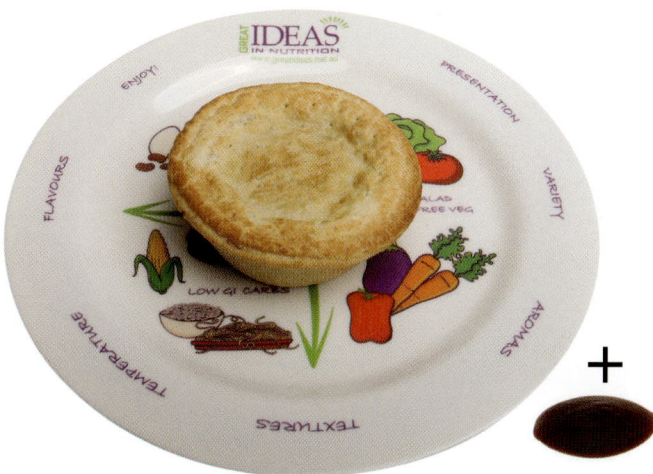

LUNCH | 107

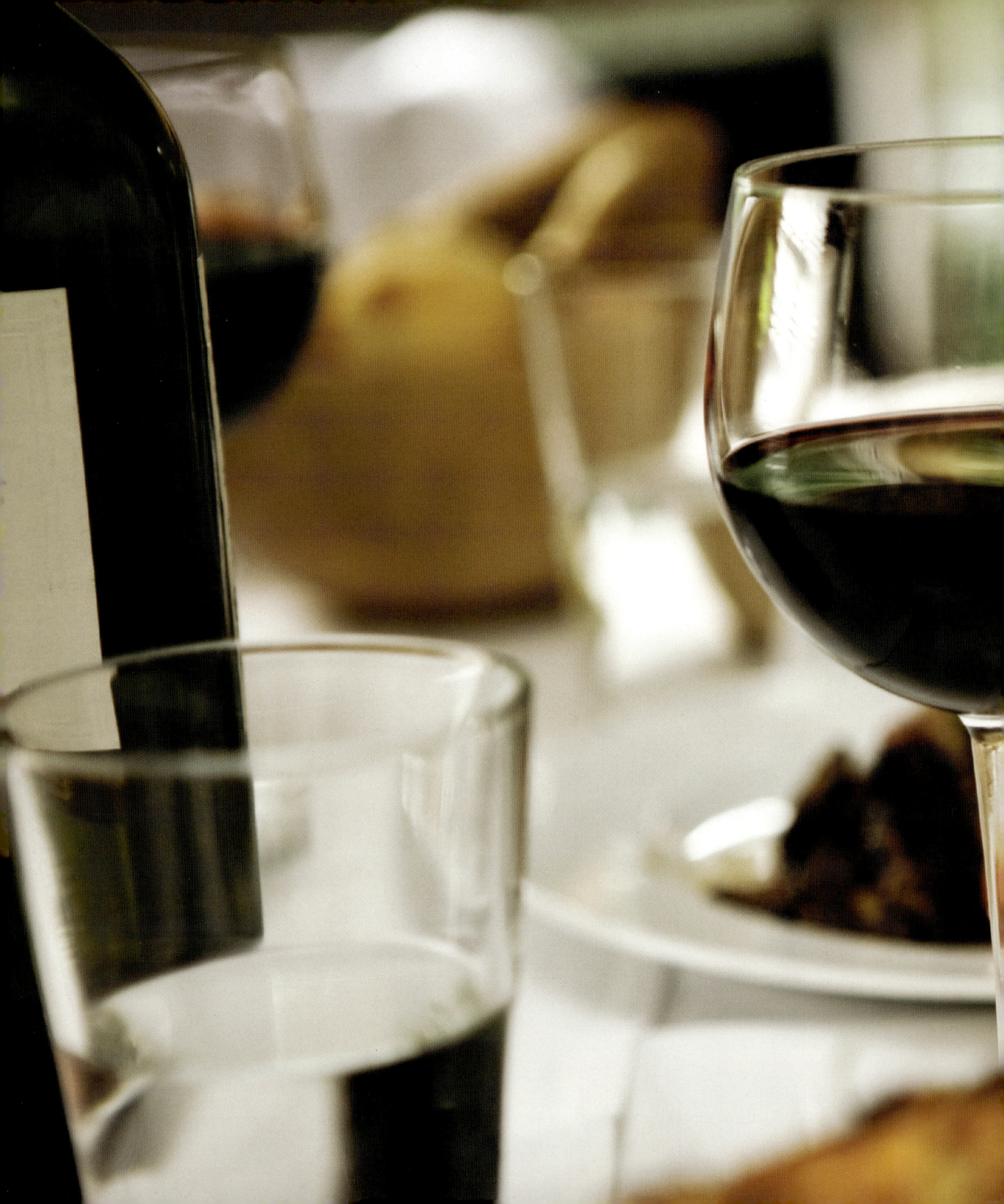

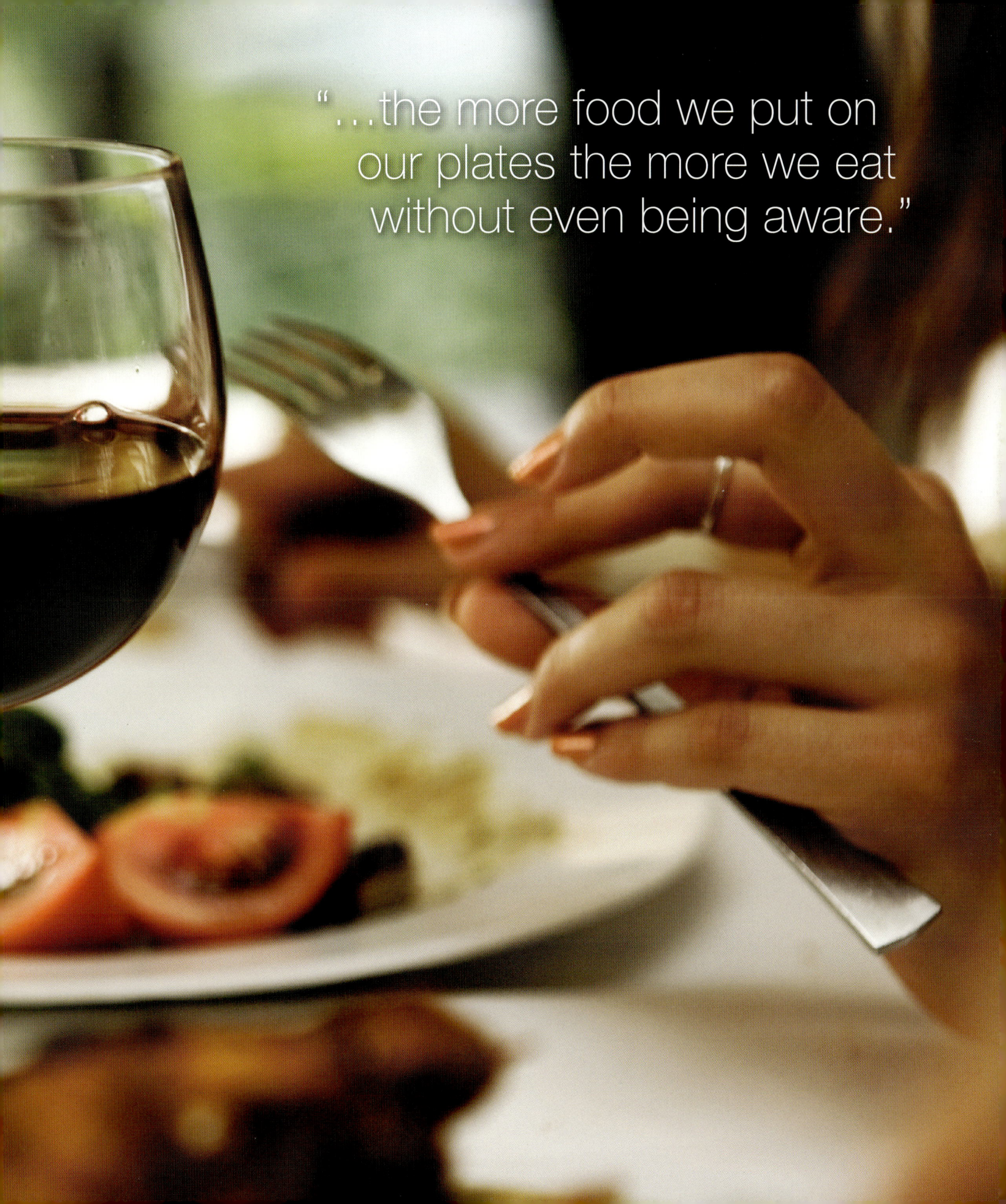

"...the more food we put on our plates the more we eat without even being aware."

CHAPTER 9

dinner

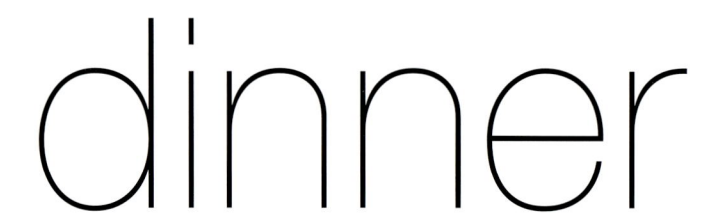

Lunches and dinners have the same number of Calories here, so you can also choose any lunch option for your evening meal.

The carbohydrate portion of the plate and the meat section contribute equal Calories. For example on the 350 Calorie / 1470 kJ portion, the meat contributes approx. 150 Calories / 630 kJ, the carbohydrate 150 Calories / 630 kJ, the 1 tablespoon of low-fat sauce or dressing contributes approx 20 Calories / 85 kJ, and the half-plate of free vegetables provides approximately 30 Calories / 125 kJ.

Using healthy cookbooks like the *4 Week Weight Loss Menu Plan*, is a great way to maintain motivation for healthy eating. Choose cookbooks with pictures for inspiration. Look for cookbooks that display the nutritional information of the recipe so you can judge the appropriateness of the serve to your needs. Note the Calorie distribution for each segment of the plate for both the larger and smaller serve:

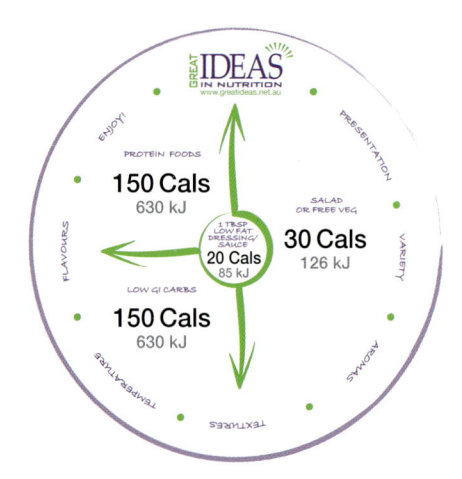

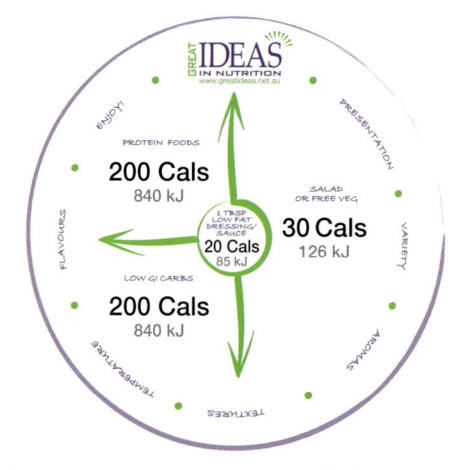

Small serve = approx 350 Cals / 1470 kJ   **Large serve = approx 450 Cals** / 1890 kJ

In effect the majority of the Calories are served on half of the plate, so if in doubt, serve only half a plate of a low-fat mixed dish and ½ a plate of salad or free veg.

Many recipes don't provide for all the segments of the meal, for example the recipe may just be for a meat curry so it won't incorporate sufficient free vegetables. You may need to plan ahead and ensure you incorporate these independently of the recipe.

110 | DINNER

CHAPTER 9

There is no standardisation for serving sizes with recipes, so the *4 Week Weight Loss Menu Plan* is an easy way to get the portion sizes right. For your own favourite recipes, check the Calorie content pertaining to each component of the meal to see how it matches the plan laid out above. Even very healthy meals can result in weight gain if served in excessive portion sizes.

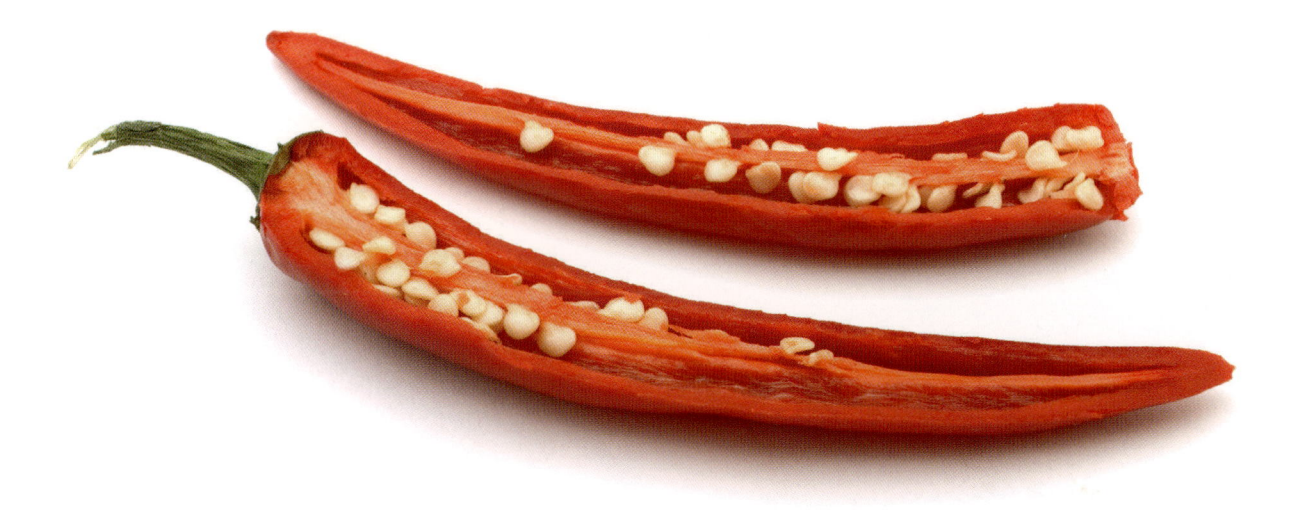

everyday menu

Curry/casserole & rice............................ 112
Mexican... 113
Stir-fry... 114
Pasta... 115
Ravioli... 116
Roast 117
Steak/seafood/chicken & salad/veg.......... 118

occasional menu

Quiche/Pie.. 123
Takeaway Asian foods 124
Pizza 125
Finger food with drinks 126
Desserts (everyday and occasional) 127
See occasional lunches for additional options

Add your own favourites by calculating the appropriate serve from Allan Borushek's *The CalorieKing Calorie Fat and Carbohydrate Counter* or apps CalorieKing or My Fitness Pal.

DINNER | 111

everyday dinner
curry/casserole & rice

Look for recipes that limit added fats to 1 tsp per serve (oil/butter/coconut milk/sour cream). Try substituting fat free evaporated milk or low-fat natural yoghurt where possible. Consider adding coconut essence to substitute for coconut milk for coconut curries. Choose basmati rice as it has a lower glycemic index (GI) or long grain brown rice.

Dhal, cucumber raita and other dishes can count as either protein or carbohydrate.

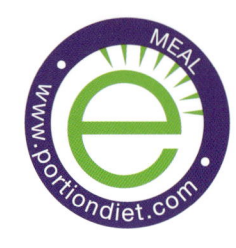

350 Calories / 1470 kJ

Small serve – ¾ cup curry/casserole protein portion (150 Cals / 630 kJ)
+ ¾ cup brown rice (150 Cals / 630 kJ)
+ 1½ cups free vegetables (30 Cals / 125 kJ)

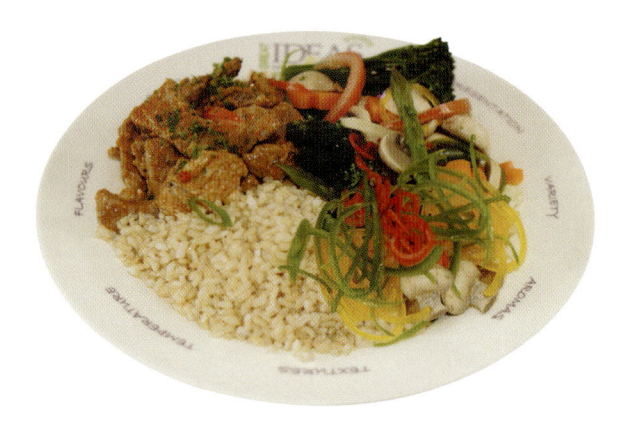

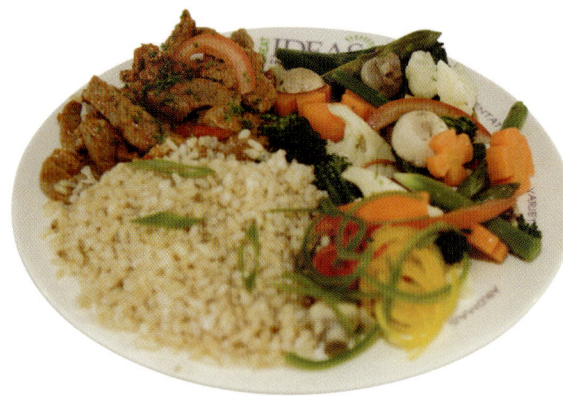

450 Calories / 1890 kJ

Large serve – 1 cup curry/casserole protein portion (200 Cals / 840 kJ)
+ 1 cup brown rice (200 Cals / 840 kJ)
+ 2 cups free vegetables (30 Cals / 125 kJ)

550 Calories / 2310 kJ

Large serve as above (450 Cals / 1890 kJ)
+ 1 Add On, (100 Cals / 420 kJ)
e.g., 6.7 fl oz / 200 ml glass of soy milk

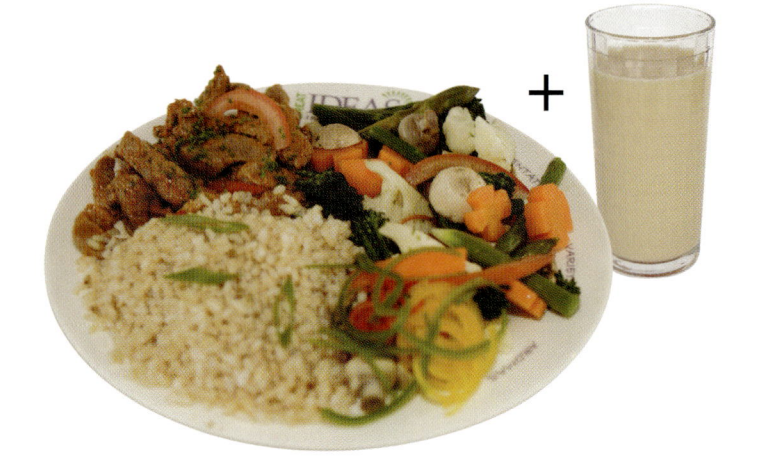

everyday dinner

mexican

Use meat, chicken or beans for the protein component, a taco shell for carbohydrate, and then some cheese can use up some of the Calories of either protein or carbs. Ensure there's a significant serve of salad. The components to watch are sour cream, avocado and cheese: ensure these are in controlled amounts.

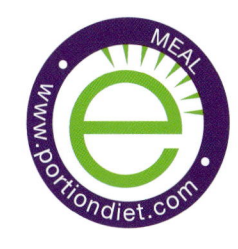

350 Calories / 1470 kJ

Small serve – 1 soft or jumbo hard taco shell (100 Cals / 420 kJ)
+ ¾ cup lean mince mix (150 Cals / 630 kJ)
+ 1½ cups salad (30 Cals / 125 kJ)
+ 0.7 fl oz / 20 ml taco sauce (20 Cals / 85 kJ)
+ 0.5 oz / 15 g grated cheese (50 Cals / 210 kJ)

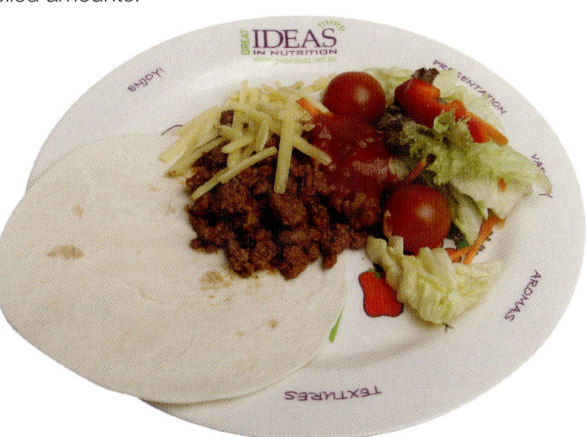

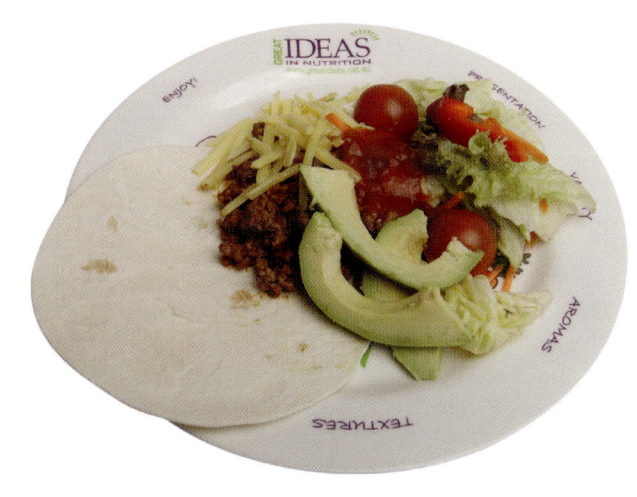

450 Calories / 1890 kJ

Large serve – 1 soft or jumbo hard taco shell (100 Cals / 420 kJ)
+ ¾ cup lean mince mix (150 Cals / 630 kJ)
+ 1½ cups salad (30 Cals / 125 kJ)
+ 0.7 fl oz / 20 ml taco sauce (20 Cals / 85 kJ)
+ 0.5 oz / 15 g grated cheese (50 Cals / 210 kJ)
+ 1 Add On e.g., ⅓ avocado (100 Cals / 420 kJ)

550 Calories / 2310 kJ

1 soft or jumbo hard taco shell (100 Cals / 420 kJ)
+ 1 cup lean mince mix (150 Cals / 630 kJ)
+ 1½ cups salad (30 Cals / 125 kJ)
+ 0.7 fl oz / 20 ml taco sauce (20 Cals / 85 kJ)
+ 1 oz / 30 g grated cheese (100 Cals / 420 kJ)
+ 1 Add On e.g., ⅓ avocado
+ 0.7 fl oz / 20 ml sour lite cream (40 Cals / 168 kJ)

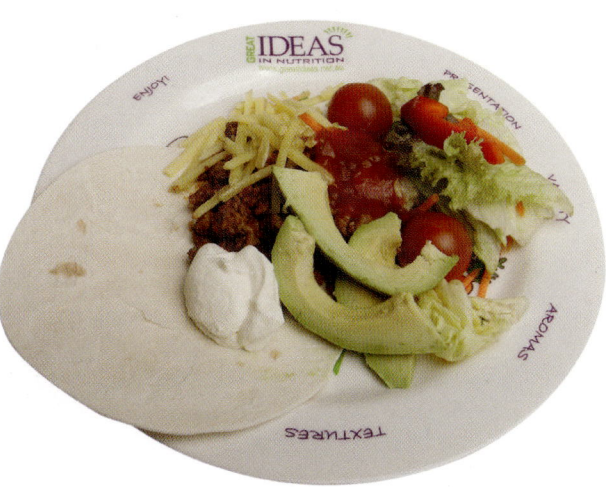

everyday dinner

stir fry

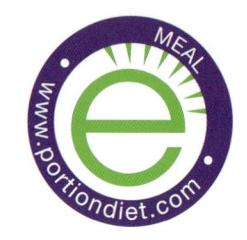

You may choose to cook and serve the components of the meal separately or in one pan or wok. If cooking in one batch it is important to get the components of the meal in the right proportion before cooking. For example, combine double the quantity of vegetables to meat and serve over ¾ of your plate, accompanied by ¼ plate of noodles or rice. Alternatively include the noodles/rice in the mix as ¼ the total volume and fill your plate to the appropriate portion size with the mixed meal.

350 Calories / 1470 kJ

Small serve – 3 oz / 90 g stir fried chicken (150 Cals / 630 kJ)
+ ¾ cup rice noodles (150 Cals / 630 kJ)
+ 1½ cups stir fried vegetables (30 Cals / 125 kJ)
+ 0.7 fl oz / 20 ml stir-fry sauce (20 Cals / 85 kJ)
per serve

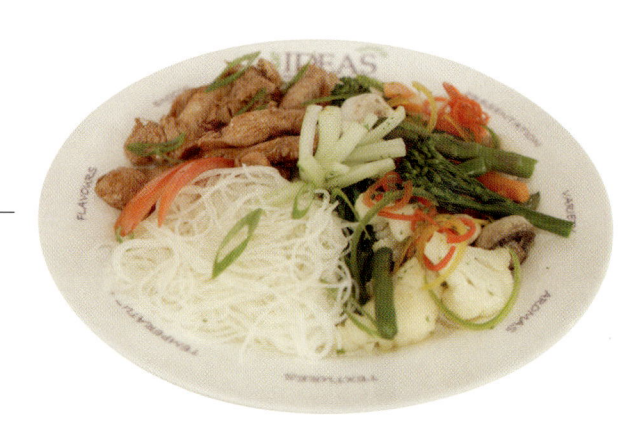

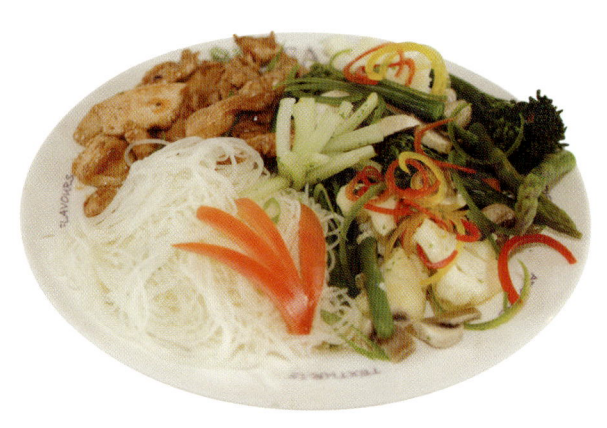

450 Calories / 1890 kJ

Large serve – 4 oz / 120 g stir fried chicken (200 Cals / 840 kJ)
+ 1 cup rice noodles (200 Cals / 840 kJ)
+ 2 cups stir fried vegetables (30 Cals / 125 kJ)
+ 0.7 fl oz / 20 ml stir fry sauce (20 Cals / 85 kJ)
per serve

550 Calories / 2310 kJ

Large serve as above (450 Cals / 1890 kJ)
+ 1 Add On food (100 Cals / 420 kJ),
e.g., 3.3 oz / 100 g yoghurt

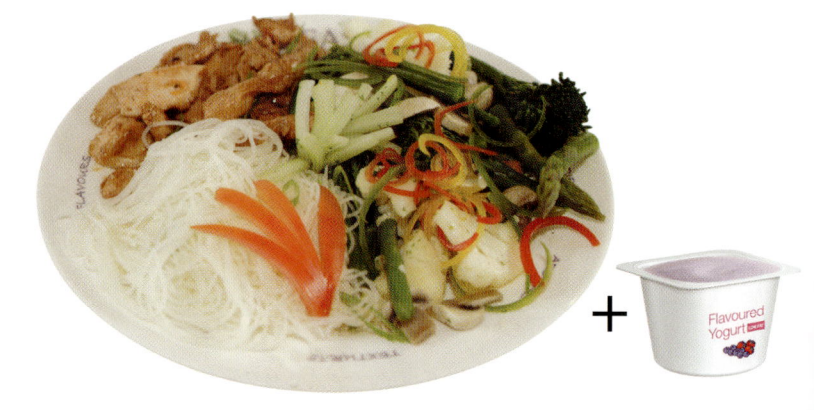

everyday dinner

pasta

Plan for equal quantities of pasta and protein and half a plate of salad. Add just a sprinkle of parmesan. Use only the leanest mince. All pastas are nutritionally similar, so it doesn't matter what shape you choose. Go for low-fat sauces, such as those with a tomato base, or use fat free evaporated milk to make a creamy sauce.

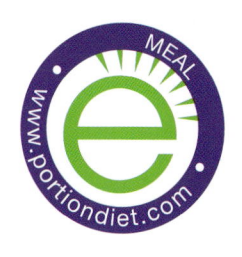

350 Calories / 1470 kJ

Small serve – ¾ cup mince (150 Cals / 630 kJ)
+ ¾ cup pasta (150 Cals / 630 kJ)
+ 1½ cups salad (30 Cals / 125 kJ)
+ 2 tsp parmesan (20 Cals / 85 kJ)

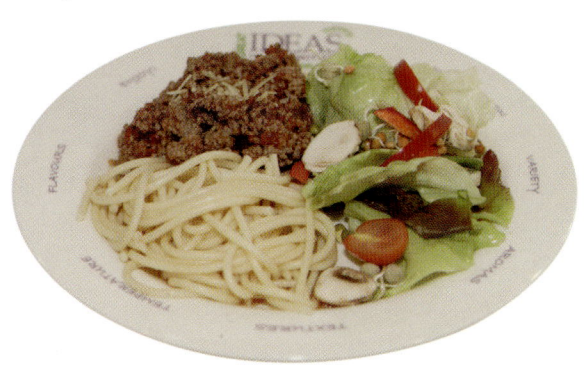

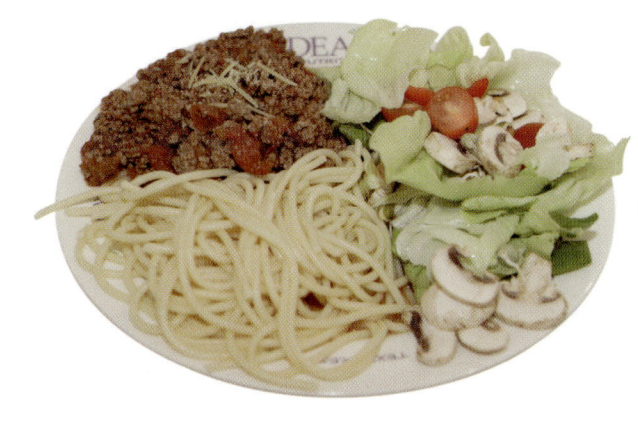

450 Calories / 1890 kJ

Large serve – 1 cup mince (200 Cals / 840 kJ)
+ 1 cup pasta (200 Cals / 840 kJ)
+ 2 cups salad (30 Cals / 125 kJ)
+ 2 tsp parmesan (20 Cals / 85 kJ)

550 Calories / 2310 kJ

Large serve as above
(450 Cals / 1890 kJ)
+ 1 Add On (100 Cals / 420 kJ),
e.g., 1 cup fruit salad

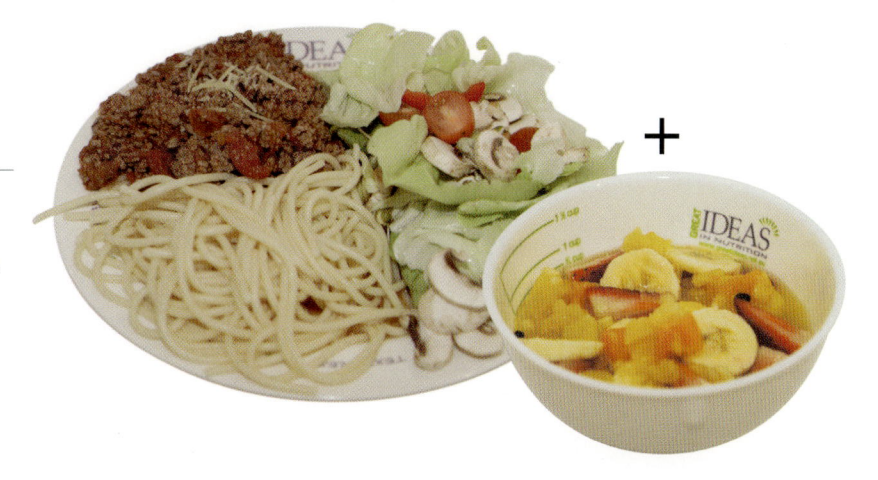

TIP Limit bacon to a hint of flavour. It's okay to use a bottled tomato pasta sauce – the redder it is, the more certain you can be that there is no cream added. For ravioli or cannelloni serve half the plate 2 cm deep with the pasta, and filling mix, and half the plate with salad (see over for example). Use oil-free dressing on the salad.

DINNER | 115

everyday dinner

ravioli

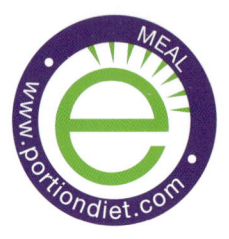

When serving a dish that is a mix of both carbohydrate and protein, or even if it is all protein or all carbohydrate (such as fish and salad or risotto) you can achieve the right Calories by filling half your plate with the dish and half with salad or free vegetables. Ravioli is used as the example here.

350 Calories / 1470 kJ

Small serve – 1½ cups ravioli in a light sauce (320 Cals / 1344 kJ)
+ 1½ cups salad (30 Cals / 125 kJ)

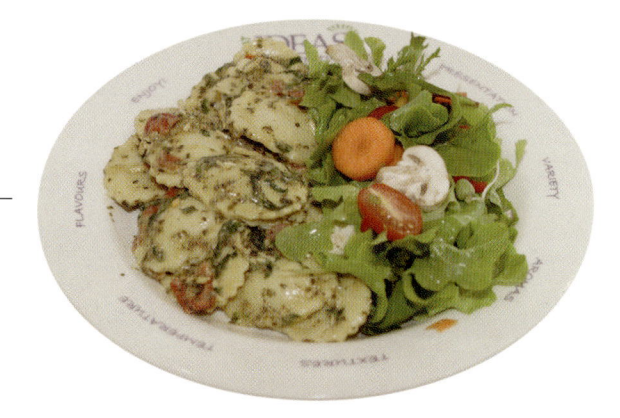

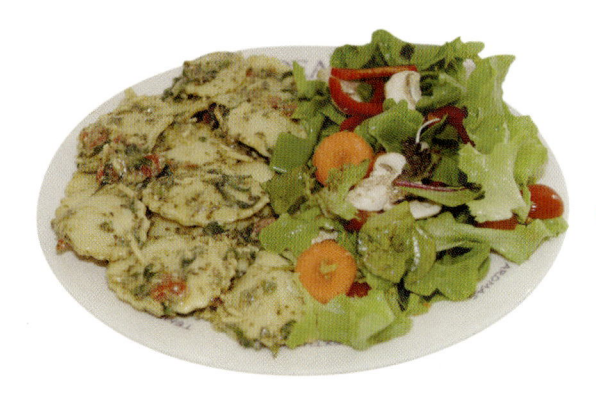

450 Calories / 1890 kJ

Large serve – 2 cups ravioli in a light sauce (420 Cals / 1764 kJ)
+ 2 cups salad (30 Cals / 125 kJ)

550 Calories / 2310 kJ

Large serve as above (450 Cals / 1890 kJ)
+ 1 extra or snack food (100 Cals / 420 kJ)
e.g., frozen yoghurt, 1 scoop 1.5 oz / 45 g

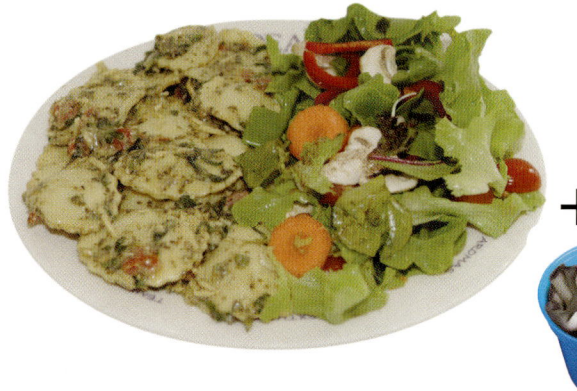

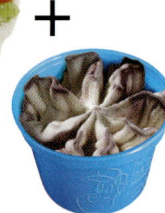

everyday dinner
roast

A roast is a family favourite for many of us. We seem to like it best the way mum made it. Consider whether there are opportunities to reduce the fat content, e.g., by placing the meat on a rack for cooking so that the fat drips away, and cooking the vegetables with just a spray of oil, or at least in vegetable oil rather than in the fat from the meat. Limit gravy to a tablespoon and trim all visible fat from the meat.

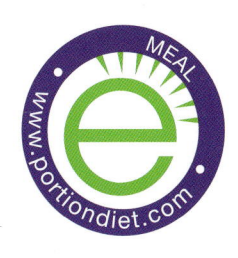

350 Calories / 1470 kJ

Small serve – 3 oz / 90 g roast meat (150 Cals / 630 kJ)
+ 3.3 oz / 100 g roast vegetables (150 Cals / 630 kJ)
+ 1½ cups free veg (30 Cals / 125 kJ)
+ 0.7 fl oz / 20 ml gravy (20 Cals / 85 kJ)

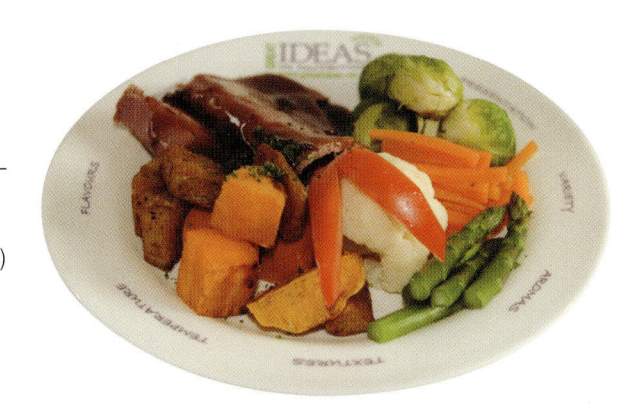

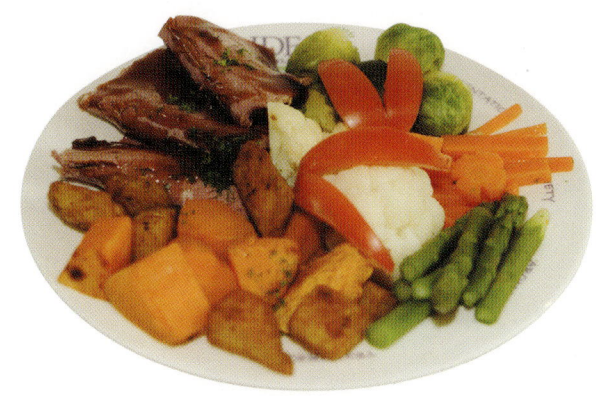

450 Calories / 1890 kJ

Large serve – 4 oz / 120 g roast meat (200 Cals / 840 kJ)
+ 4.7 oz / 140 g roast vegetables (200 Cals / 840 kJ)
+ 2 cups free vegetables (30 Cals / 125 kJ)
+ 0.7 fl oz / 20 ml gravy (20 Cals / 85 kJ)

550 Calories / 2310 kJ

Large serve as above (450 Cals / 1890 kJ)
+ 1 Add On e.g., ½ cup low fat pudding (100 Cals / 420 kJ)

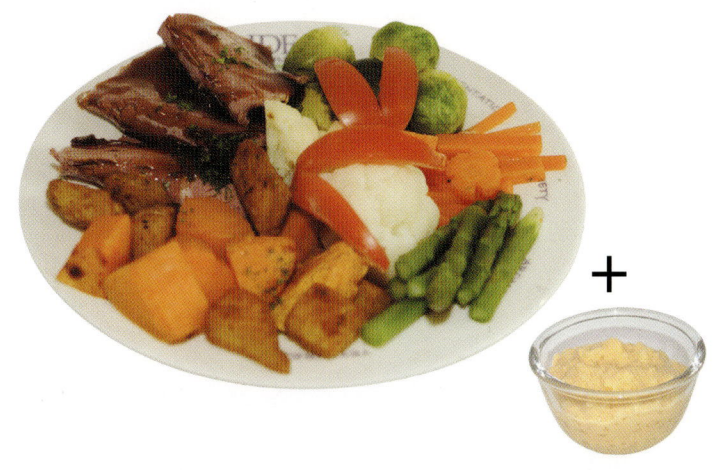

TIP Remember that as the fat content of the food increases you will need to decrease the portion size of that meal component. The way the starchy vegetables are baked will determine how small that segment of the plate should really be. If they are cooked with just a spray of oil, fill the plate as designed.

everyday dinner
steak/seafood/chicken & salad/veg

No matter what type of meat you choose, it is perfect for the plate. Your starchy section could be filled with any of the choices discussed earlier. Then vary between salad or vegetables for the vegetables component and a variety of sauces for an endless array of dishes.

350 Calories / 1470 kJ

Small serve – 3 oz / 90 g cooked protein portion (150 Cals / 630 kJ)
+ ¾ cup couscous (150 Cals / 630 kJ)
+ 1½ cups salad (30 Cals / 125 kJ)
+ 0.7 fl oz / 20 ml 'No oil' salad dressing (20 Cals / 85 kJ)

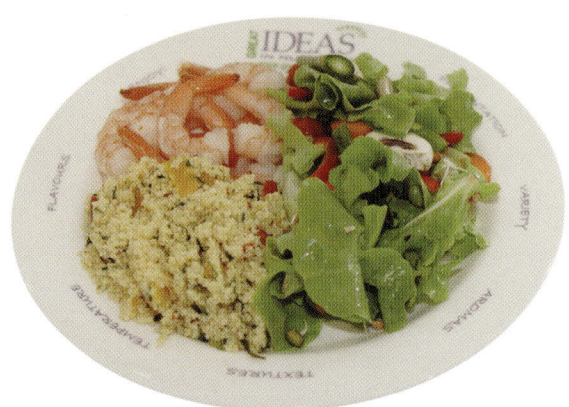

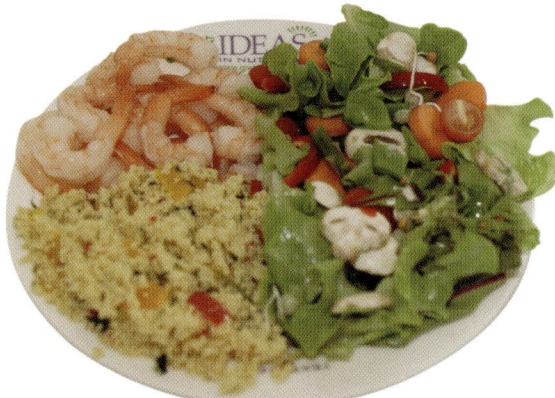

450 Calories / 1890 kJ

Large serve – 4 oz / 120 g cooked protein portion (200 Cals / 840 kJ)
+ 1 cup couscous (200 Cals / 840 kJ)
+ 2 cups salad (30 Cals / 125 kJ)
+ 0.7 fl oz / 20 ml 'No oil' dressing (20 Cals / 85 kJ)

550 Calories / 2310 kJ

Large serve as above (450 Cals / 1890 kJ)
+ 1 Add On e.g., 14 cashew nuts added to the salad (100 Cals / 420 kJ)

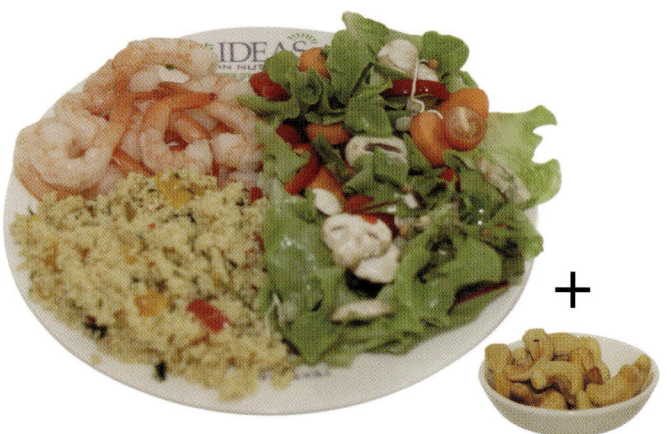

TIP Trim visible fat from meat and remove skin from chicken.
When no drink is shown, only an item from the free foods list can be added to the meal. Water can be added in unlimited amounts.

everyday dinner

steak/seafood/chicken & salad/veg continued

A note on sausages

Sausages are a popular and convenient meat for outdoor cooking. The fat content of sausages varies but would be too high to be considered an everyday option. Reduced fat sausages usually contain 8 g fat per 100 g compared to 4 g per 100 g in lean red meat, so while they are higher in saturated fats, they could be considered an acceptable everyday choice.

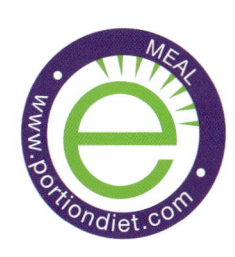

350 Calories / 1470 kJ

Small serve – 1 reduced fat sausage (150 Cals / 630 kJ)
+ ¾ cup of mashed sweet potato (150 Cals / 630 kJ)
+ 1½ cups free vegetables (30 Cals / 125 kJ)

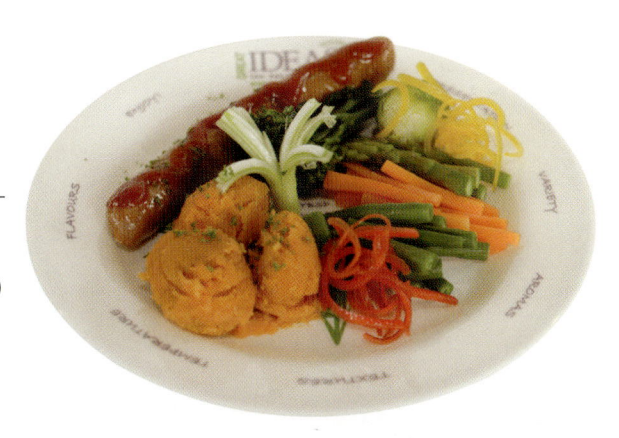

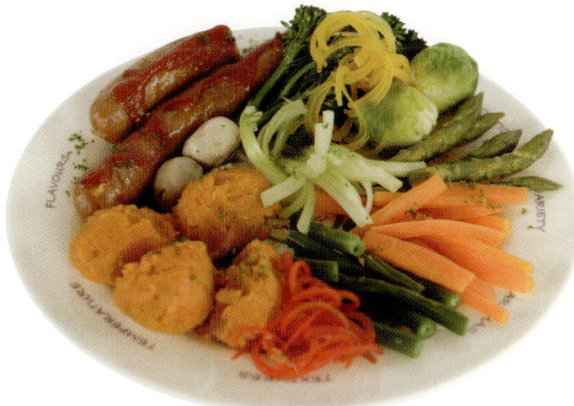

450 Calories / 1890 kJ

Large serve – 1½ reduced fat sausages (200 Cals / 840 kJ)
+ 1 cup mashed sweet potato (200 Cals / 840 kJ)
+ 2 cups free vegetables (30 Cals / 125 kJ)
+ 1 tsp oil (20 Cals / 85 kJ)

550 Calories / 2310 kJ

Large serve as above (450 Cals / 1890 kJ)
+ 1 Add On e.g., glass of reduced fat milk (100 Cals / 420 kJ)

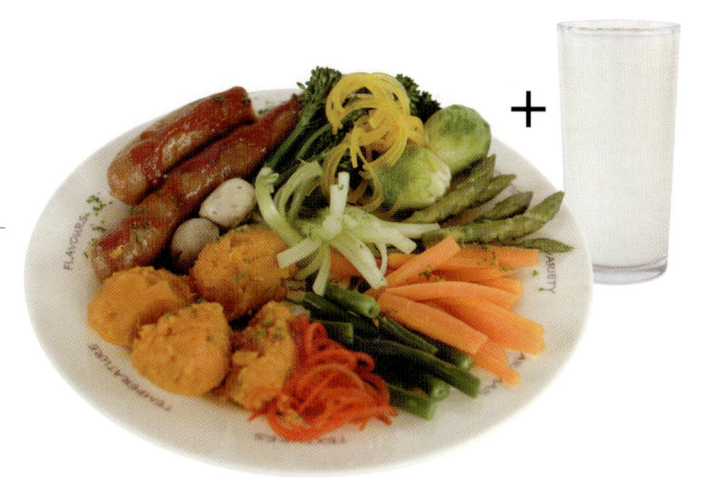

Continued over ❯

DINNER | 119

everyday dinner

steak/seafood/chicken & salad/veg continued

A note on vegetarian dishes

Vegetarian options substitute very well for animal protein. The plate portions are correct for tofu, beans and lentils. Here we have used lentil patties.

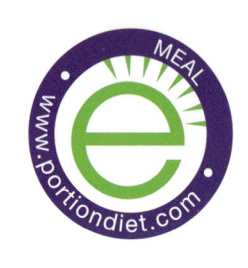

350 Calories / 1470 kJ

Small serve – 1 lentil patty (150 Cals / 630 kJ)
+ 1 medium corn cob (150 Cals / 630 kJ)
+ 1½ cups vegetables (30 Cals / 125 kJ)
+ 1 tsp oil for stir frying veg (20 Cals / 85 kJ)

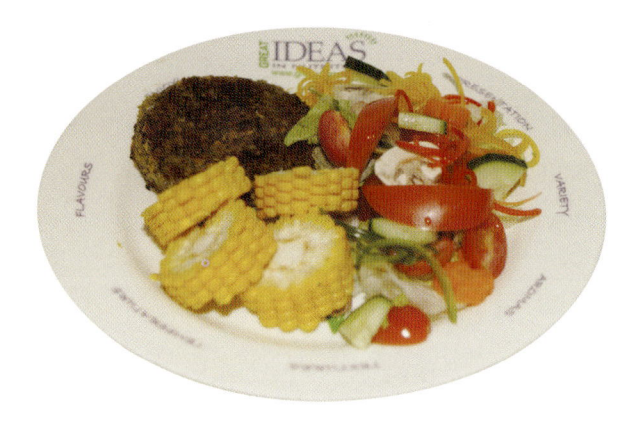

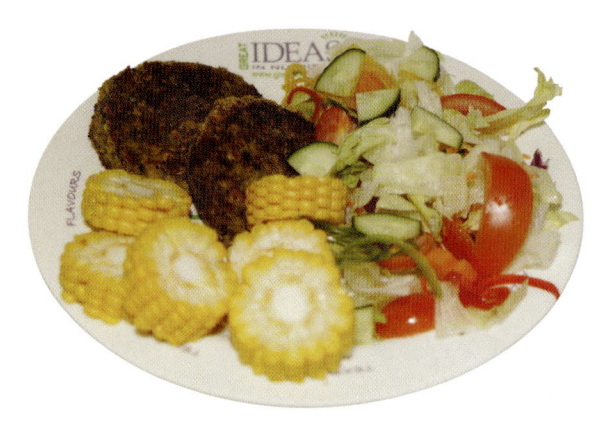

450 Calories / 1890 kJ

Large serve – 1½ lentil patties (225 Cals / 945 kJ)
+ 1 large corn cob (175 Cals / 735 kJ)
+ 2 cups free vegetables (30 Cals / 125 kJ)
+ 1 tsp oil for stir frying veg (20 Cals / 85 kJ)

550 Calories / 2310 kJ

Large serve as above (450 Cals / 1890 kJ)
+ 1 Add On e.g., 6.7 fl oz / 200 ml glass of fruit juice (100 Cals / 420 kJ)

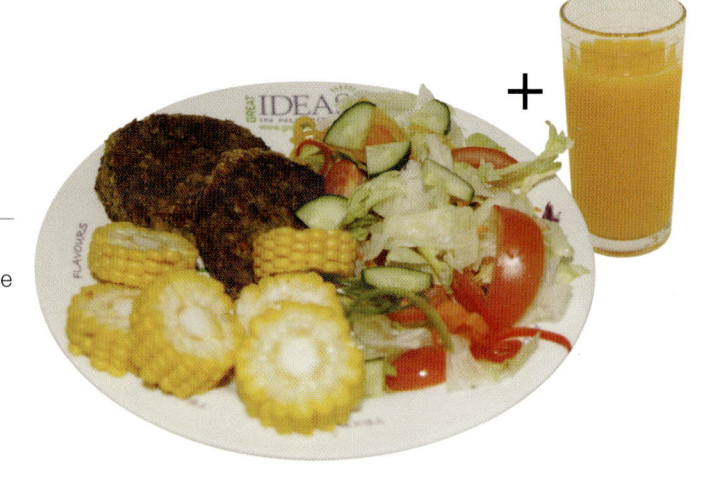

everyday dinner

steak/seafood/chicken & salad/veg continued

A note on steak dishes

When buying steak, choose cuts that enable you to easily remove the visible fat. Serve with an array of fresh or frozen vegetables and a touch of sauce.

✓ 350 Calories / 1470 kJ

Small Serve: 3 oz / 90 g cooked (4 oz / 120 g raw) steak (150 Cals / 630 kJ)
+ ¾ cup combined baby potatoes and peas (150 Cals / 630 kJ)
+ 1½ cups free vegetables (30 Cals / 125 kJ)
+ 0.7 fl oz / 20 ml steak sauce (20 Cals / 85 kJ)

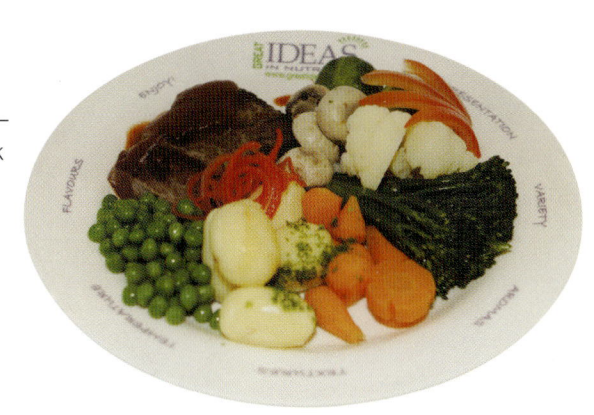

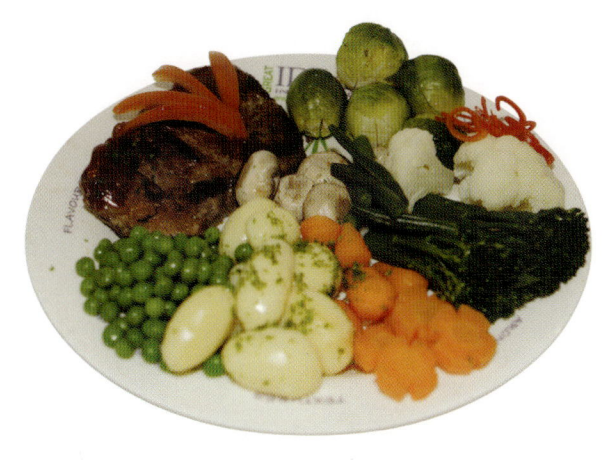

✓✓ 450 Calories / 1890 kJ

Large serve – 4 oz / 120 g cooked (5 oz / 150 g raw) steak (200 Cals / 840 kJ)
+ 1 cup combined baby potatoes and peas (200 Cals / 840 kJ)
+ 2 cups free vegetables (30 Cals / 125 kJ)
+ 0.7 fl oz / 20 ml steak sauce (20 Cals / 85 kJ)

✓ 550 Calories / 2310 kJ

Large serve as above (450 Cals / 1890 kJ)
+ 1 Add On e.g., glass of reduced fat milk (100 Cals / 420 kJ)

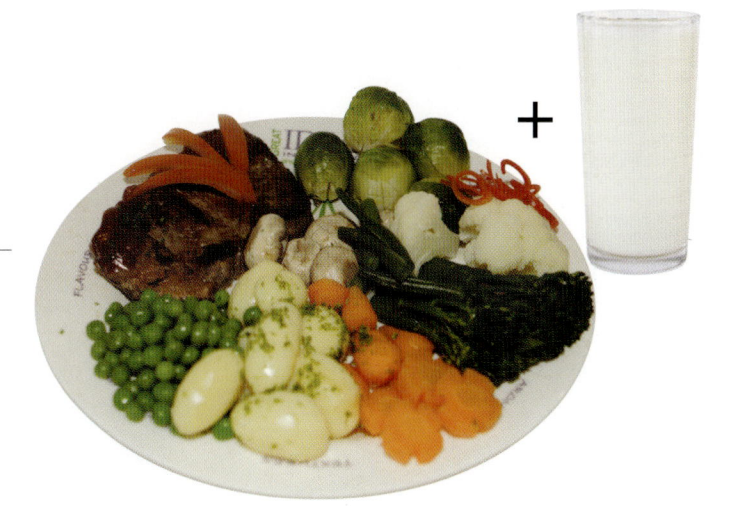

DINNER

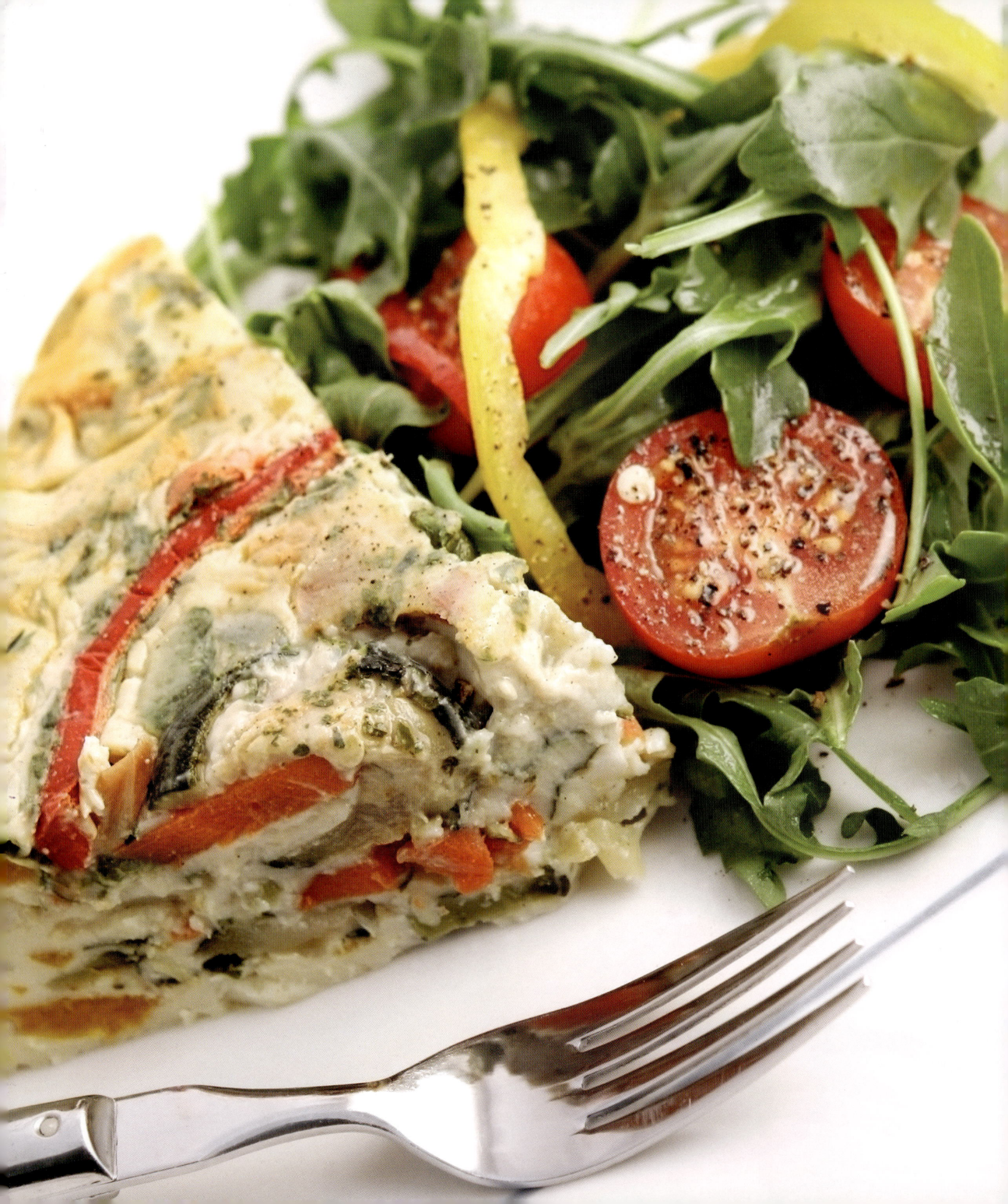

occasional dinner
quiche/pie

Pies and quiches may be 2 cm high, however, they contain much higher levels of fat than required to fit the plate model. Note the correct amounts for your calorie needs.

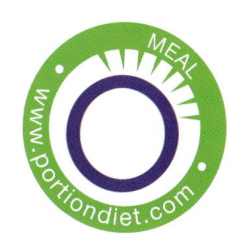

350 Calories / 1470 kJ

25% of a small quiche or pie, 4.2 oz / 125 g

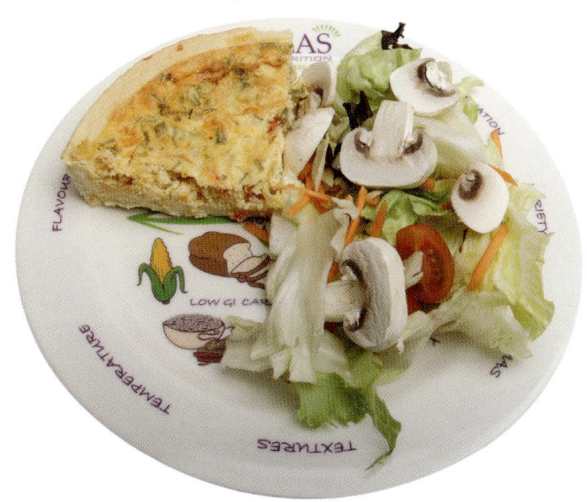

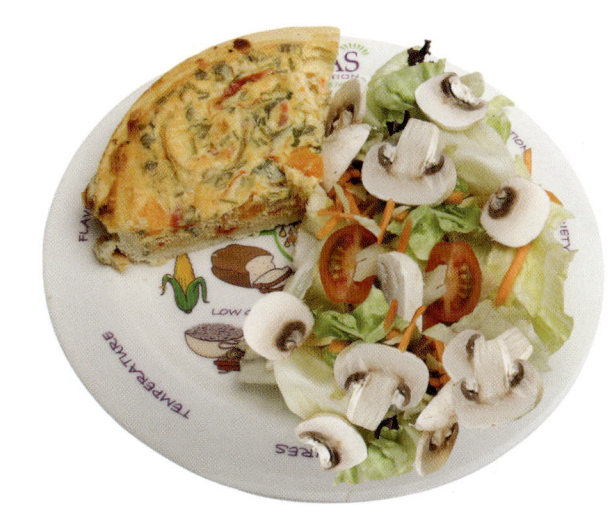

450 Calories / 1890 kJ

33% of a small quiche or pie, 5.3 oz / 160 g

550 Calories / 2310 kJ

40% of a small quiche or pie, 6.7 oz / 200 g

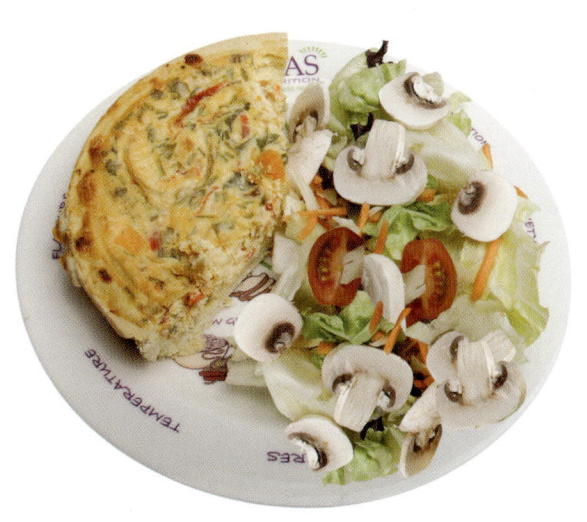

occasional dinner
takeaway asian foods

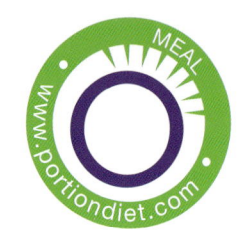

Take away Asian food ingredients are often fried before being stir fried. Choose meat and vegetable based meals rather than meat only dishes. Avoid choices with deep fried items as the appropriate portion size becomes smaller and less fulfilling. Jasmine rice is high GI, however even choosing steamed rice rather than fried rice would allow a slightly larger portion size for the Calories.

✓ **350 Calories** / 1470 kJ

Small serve – 1 cup total of mixed meat, vegetable and fried rice dishes

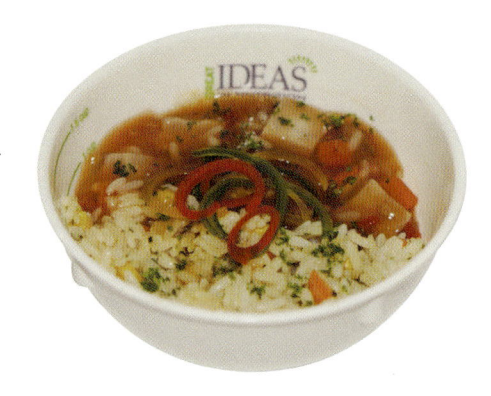

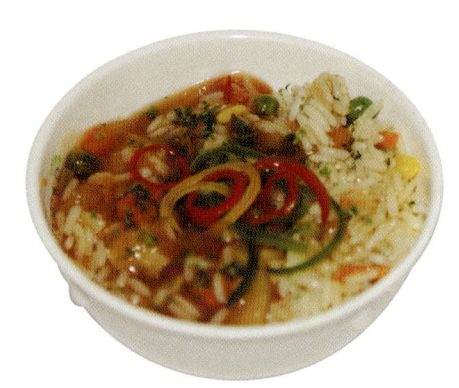

✓✓ **450 Calories** / 1890 kJ

Large serve – 1½ cups total of mixed meat, vegetable and fried rice dishes

✓ **550 Calories** / 2310 kJ

Large serve as above (450 Cals / 1890 kJ) + 1 Add On e.g., 6.7 fl oz / 200 ml soft drink

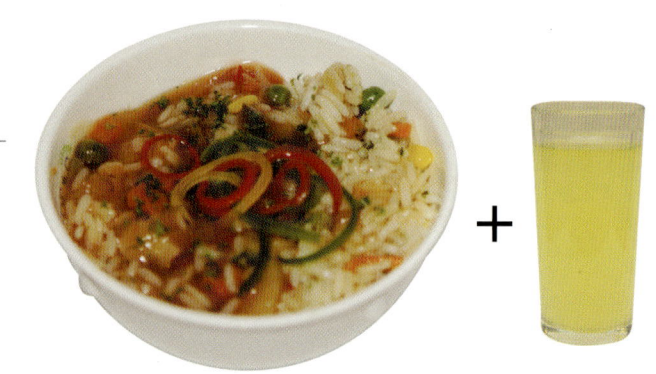

TIP A cupful of chicken and corn or long soup could substitute for the Calories of ⅓ of a cup of the meal and may be more satisfying.

occasional dinner

pizza

Choose thin and crispy styles. Avoid stuffed crusts and extra meat or cheese.

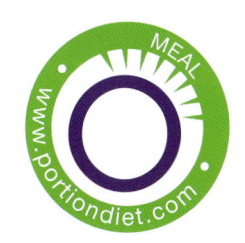

✓ **350 Calories** / 1470 kJ

Small serve – 2 slices thin crust (350 Cals / 1470 kJ)

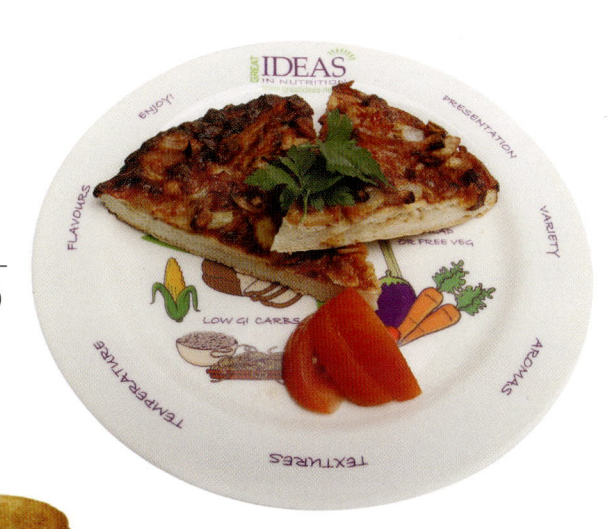

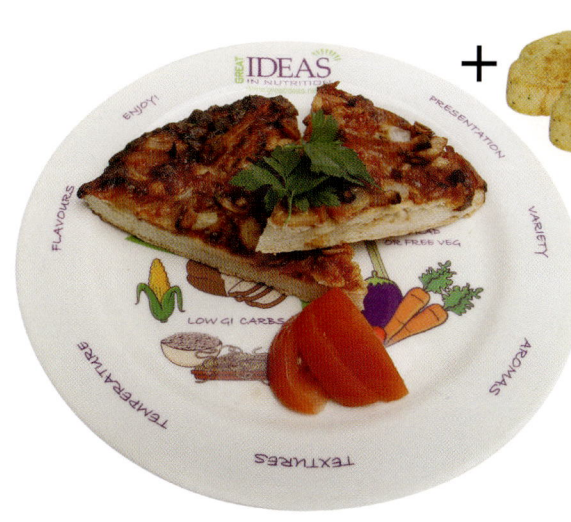

✓✓ **450 Calories** / 1890 kJ

Small serve – 2 thin slices thin crust (350 Cals / 1470 kJ) + 1 extra, e.g., 2 slices garlic bread (100 Cals / 420 kJ)

✓ **550 Calories** / 2310 kJ

3 slices thin crust (500 Cals / 2100 kJ) + ½ an extra e.g., 1 slice garlic bread (50 Cals / 210 kJ)

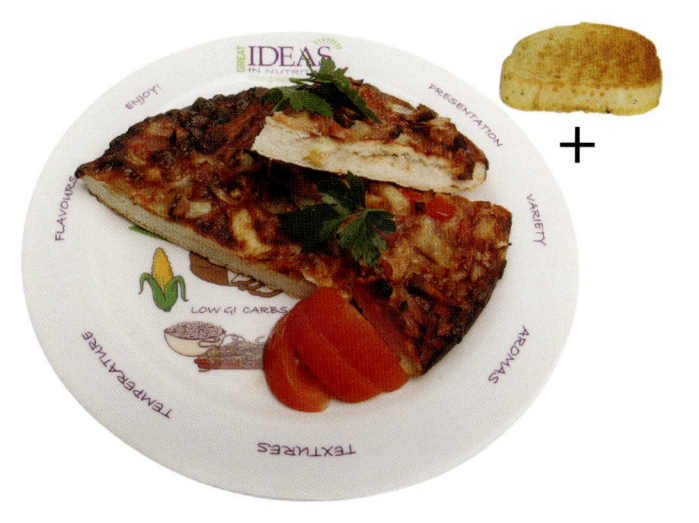

TIP If you have the opportunity to eat the pizza at home on a plate, try eating it with a knife and fork and with a half plate of salad for greater satisfaction.

DINNER | 125

occasional dinner

finger food

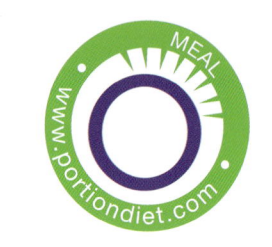

It is quite common to consume the Calories of an entire meal in finger food. See below for estimates of common intakes.

350 Calories / 1470 kJ

6 fried hors d'oeuvres (250 Cals / 1050 kJ)
+ 5 fl oz / 150 ml wine (100 Cals / 420 kJ)

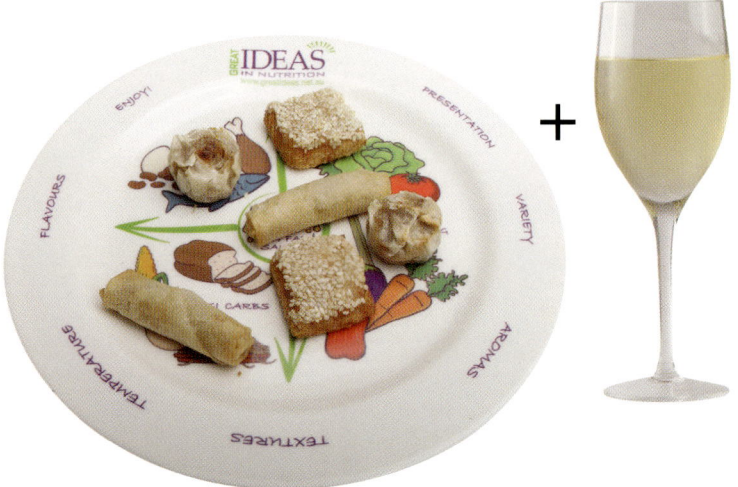

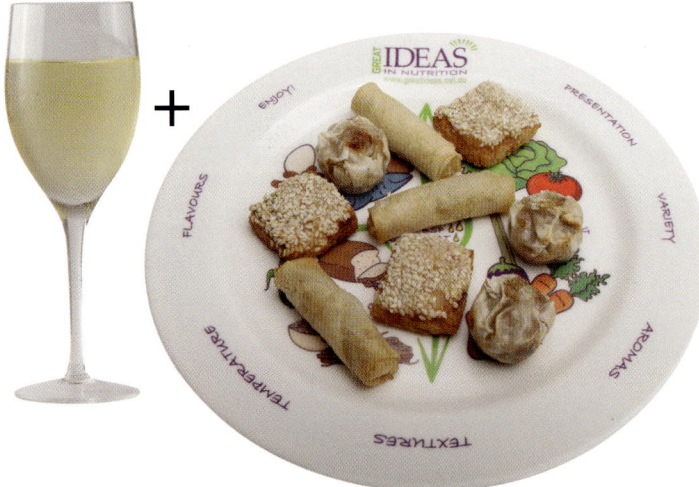

450 Calories / 1890 kJ

9 fried hors d'oeuvres (350 Cals / 1470 kJ)
+ 5 fl oz / 150 ml wine (100 Cals / 420 kJ)

550 Calories / 2310 kJ

9 fried hors d'oeuvres (350 Cals / 1470 kJ)
+ 10 fl oz / 300 ml wine (200 Cals / 840 kJ)

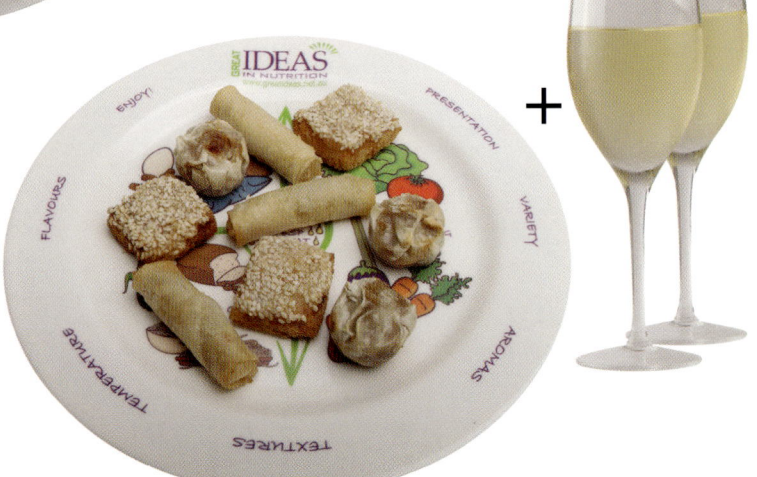

everyday dessert

desserts

If you have a sweet tooth and enjoy desserts, base them around fruit or dairy foods. Choose from the snack list for desserts. There you will find the following options and more. Wait a while after your evening meal to consume your dessert as your supper snack.

Everyday desserts/suppers/snacks (100 Cals / 420 kJ)

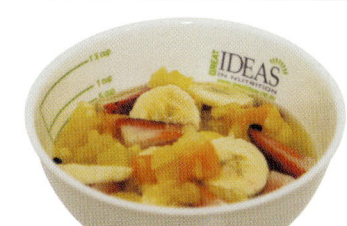

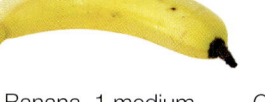

Banana, 1 medium, 5.7 oz / 170 g

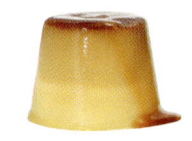

Creme Caramel / Spanish style custard, ½ cup, 4 oz / 125 g

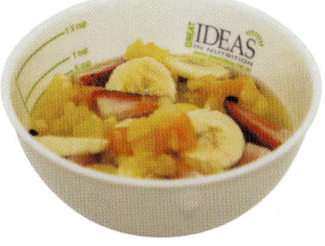

Fruit salad, 1 cup

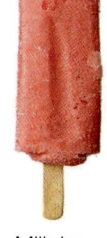

Milk ice, 2 oz / 60 g

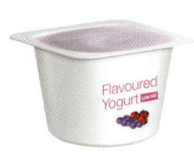

Yoghurt, regular or low fat, flavoured, 3.3 oz / 100 g

occasional dessert

Occasional desserts/suppers/snacks (100 Cals / 420 kJ)

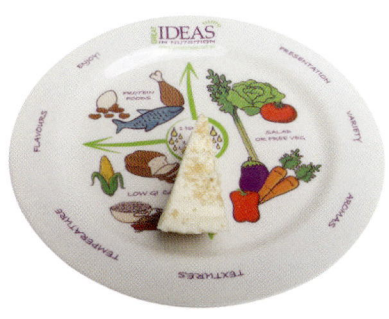

French Cream Cheesecake, 1.2 inch / 3 cm wide

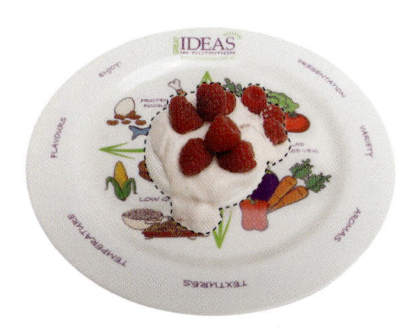

Meringue nest 0.3 oz / 10 g, low fat yoghurt 1.7 oz / 50 g + ¼ cup berries

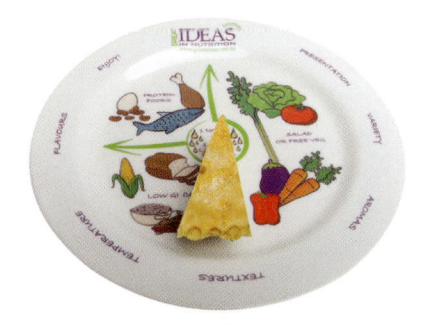

Apple Pie, 1.2 inch / 3 cm wide

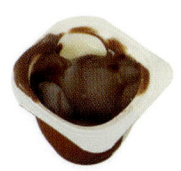

Chocolate custard, ½ cup

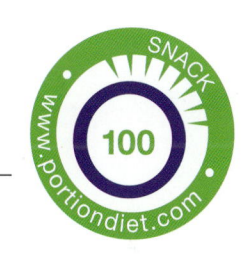

DINNER | 127

"Evidence suggests we wouldn't notice if our portion sizes decreased. What a painless method of weight control!"

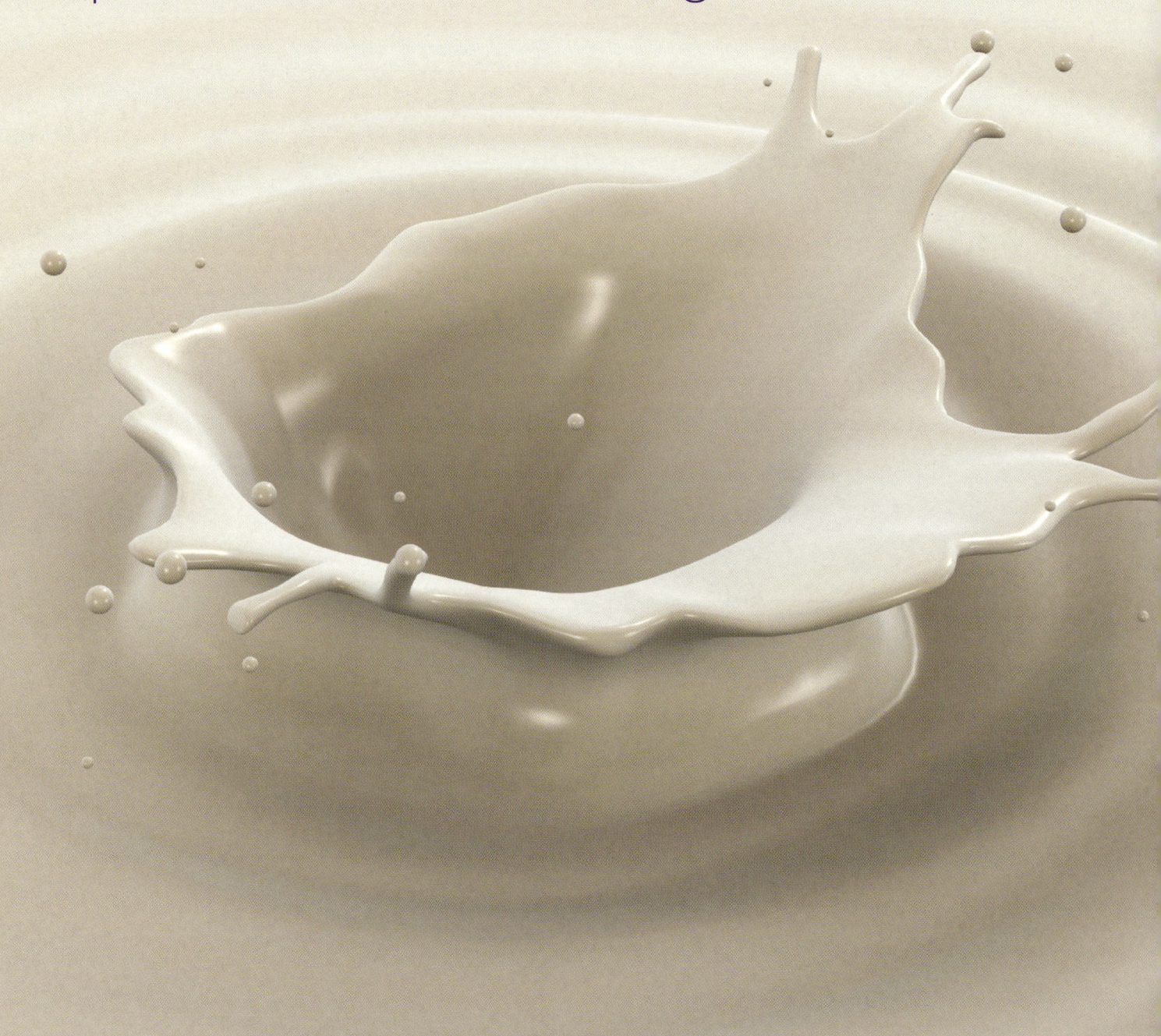

CHAPTER 10

appendices

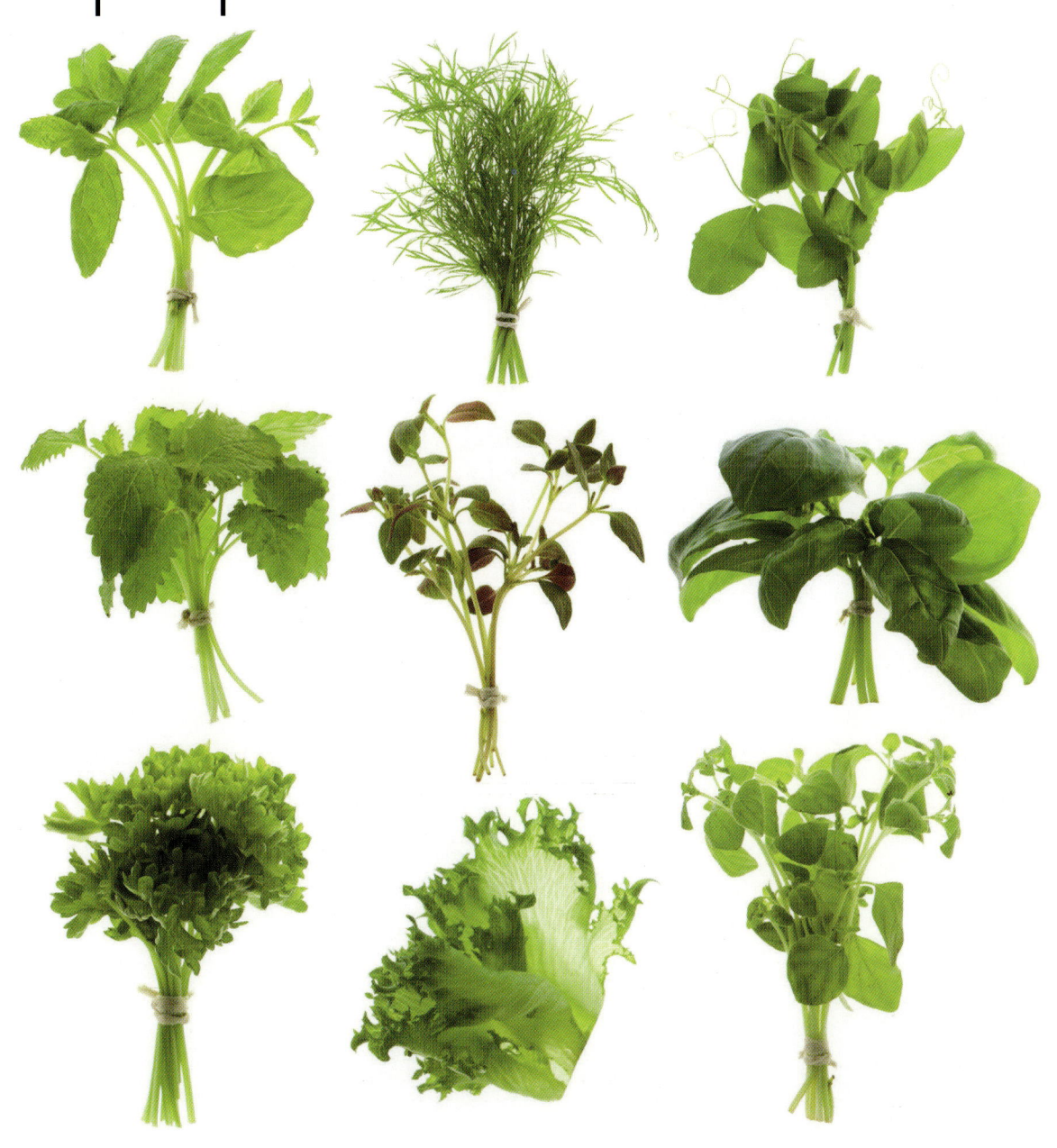

APPENDIX | 129

appendix 1

fruit

A small piece of fruit, weighing approximately 3.3 oz / 100 g equates to 50 Calories / 210 kJ. Larger serves of fruit weighing 6.7 oz / 200 g equate to 100 Calories / 420 kJ. Small pieces only are shown in this section – simply double the portion for a 100 Calorie / 420 kJ Add On or an everyday snack.

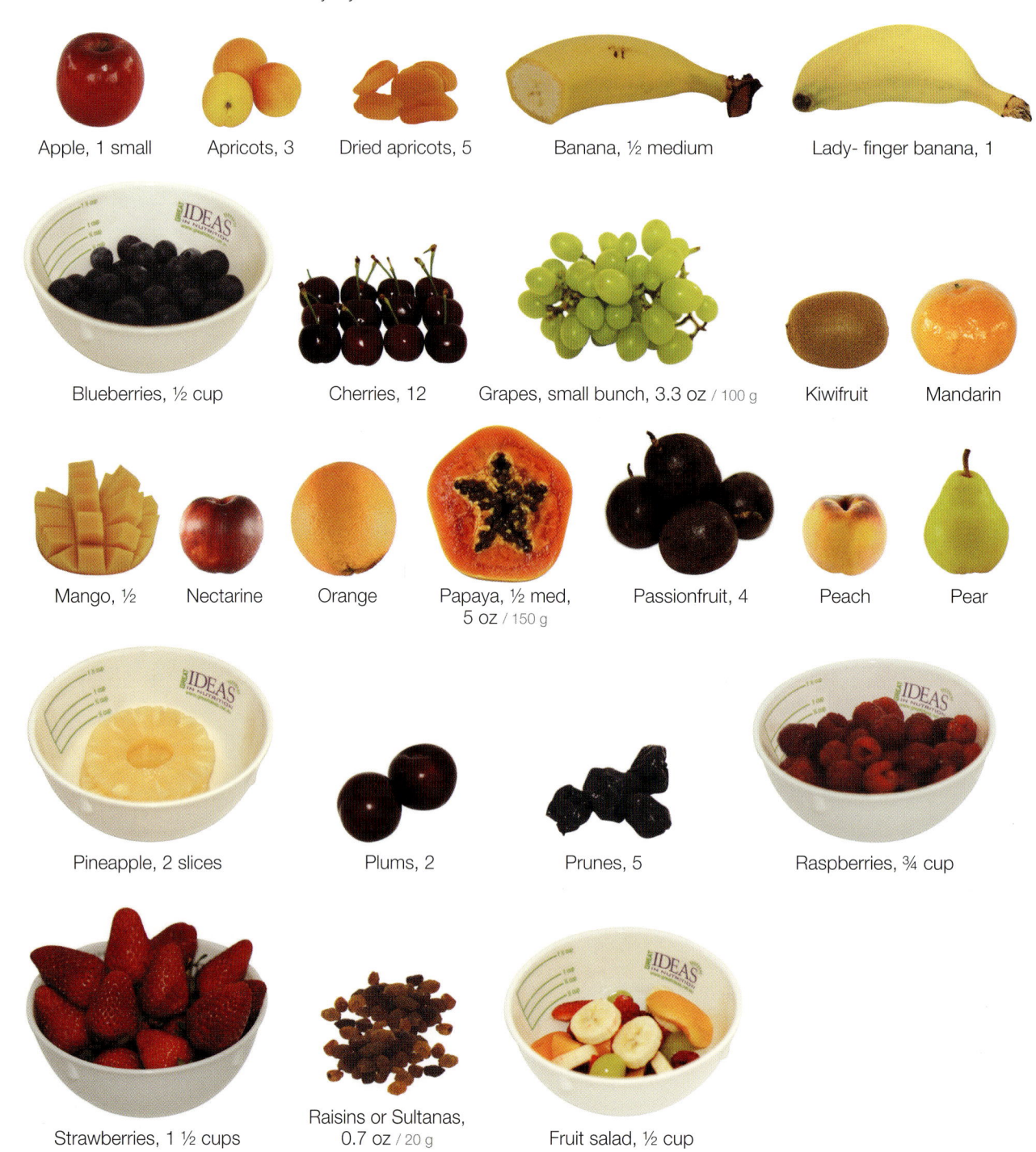

- Apple, 1 small
- Apricots, 3
- Dried apricots, 5
- Banana, ½ medium
- Lady-finger banana, 1
- Blueberries, ½ cup
- Cherries, 12
- Grapes, small bunch, 3.3 oz / 100 g
- Kiwifruit
- Mandarin
- Mango, ½
- Nectarine
- Orange
- Papaya, ½ med, 5 oz / 150 g
- Passionfruit, 4
- Peach
- Pear
- Pineapple, 2 slices
- Plums, 2
- Prunes, 5
- Raspberries, ¾ cup
- Strawberries, 1 ½ cups
- Raisins or Sultanas, 0.7 oz / 20 g
- Fruit salad, ½ cup

appendix 1
fruit

Occasional fruit (higher GI)

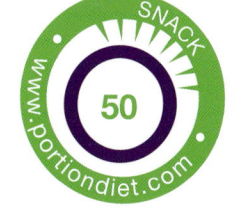

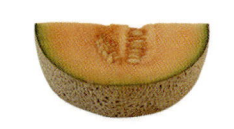

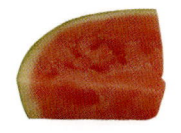

Cantaloupe / Rockmelon

Watermelon

If you prefer some more exotic fruit, check the amount for a 50 Cal / 210 kJ serve in Allan Borushek's *The CalorieKing Calorie Fat and Carbohydrate Counter* or apps CalorieKing or My Fitness Pal and record it here.

appendix 2

add ons = 100 Calories / 420 kJ

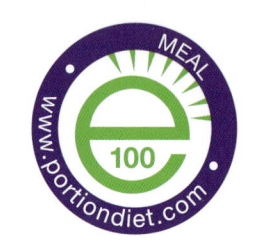

'Add ons' are foods that easily add to meals and contain approximately 100 Calories / 420 kJ. Use this section to develop your knowledge so you'll be able to look at a meal served in a café and easily 'count up' the approximate Calories so you know where to stop. Any choice from the snack list could appear here, however we have shown representative images for simplicity.

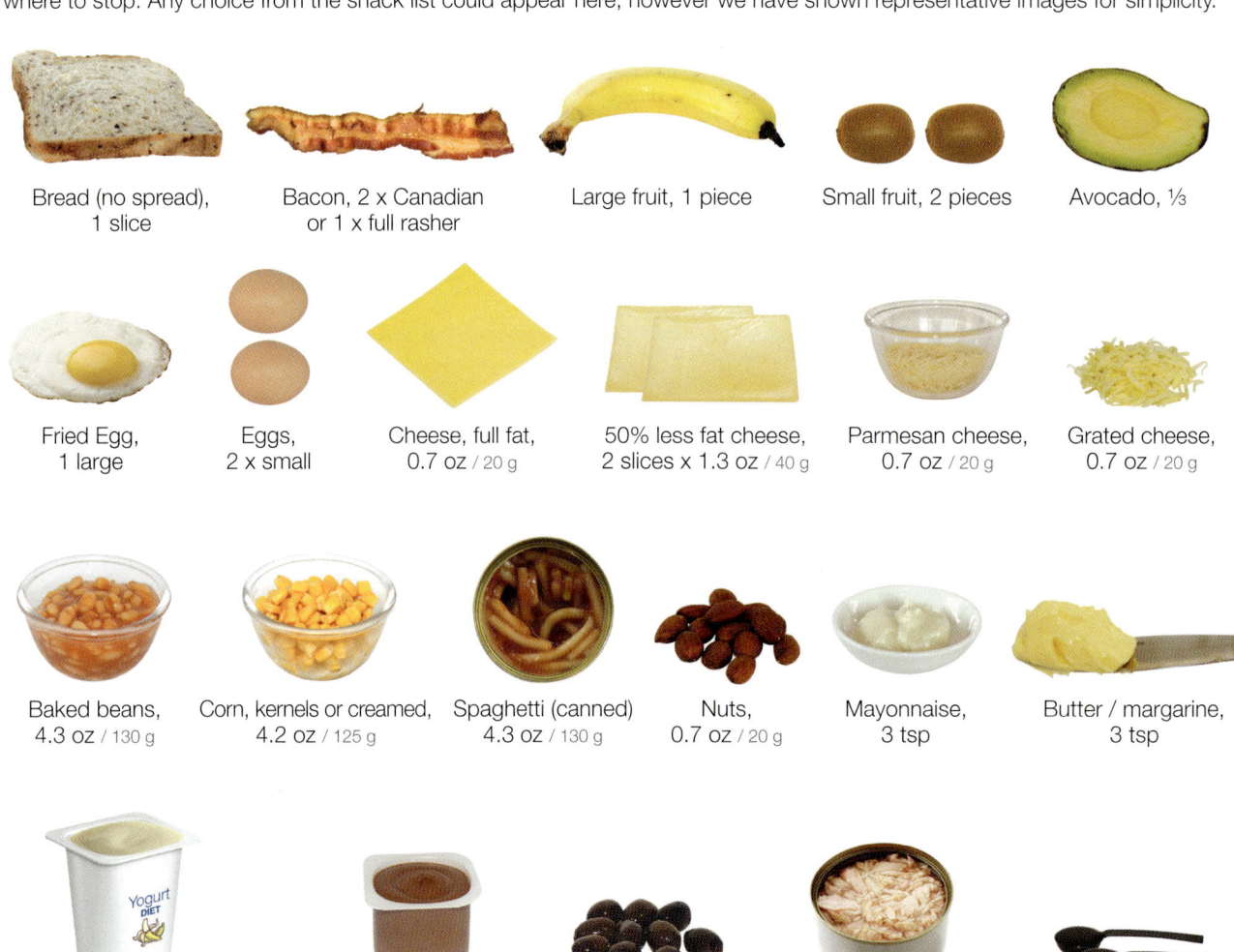

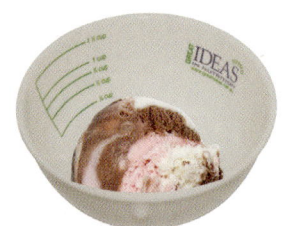

Bread (no spread), 1 slice

Bacon, 2 x Canadian or 1 x full rasher

Large fruit, 1 piece

Small fruit, 2 pieces

Avocado, ⅓

Fried Egg, 1 large

Eggs, 2 x small

Cheese, full fat, 0.7 oz / 20 g

50% less fat cheese, 2 slices x 1.3 oz / 40 g

Parmesan cheese, 0.7 oz / 20 g

Grated cheese, 0.7 oz / 20 g

Baked beans, 4.3 oz / 130 g

Corn, kernels or creamed, 4.2 oz / 125 g

Spaghetti (canned), 4.3 oz / 130 g

Nuts, 0.7 oz / 20 g

Mayonnaise, 3 tsp

Butter / margarine, 3 tsp

Yoghurt, artificially sweetened, 6.7 oz / 200 g

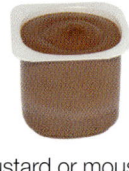

Custard or mousse, 3.3 oz / 100 g

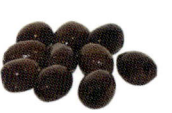

Olives, 10

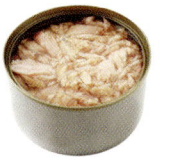

Tuna, salmon or chicken, canned, 3.7 oz / 110 g

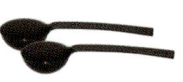

Oil, 2 tsp

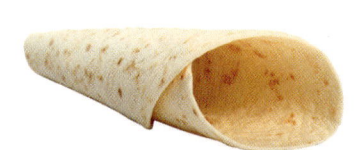

Light ice cream, various brands, 1 scoop

Tortilla, small, wholegrain, 1.3 oz / 40 g

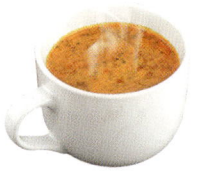

Soup in a cup, various brands, 6.7 fl oz / 200 ml

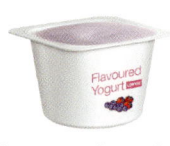

Yoghurt, regular or low fat, flavoured, 3.3 oz / 100 g

appendix 2

add ons *continued*

Occasional Add Ons

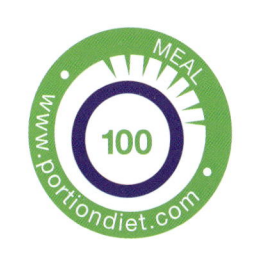

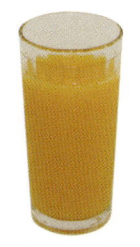

Juice, 6.7 fl oz / 200 ml

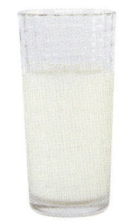

Full cream milk/soy, 5 fl oz / 150 ml

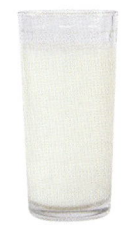

Lite milk/soy, 6.7 fl oz / 200 ml

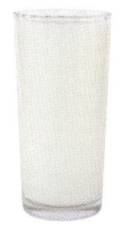

Skim milk/soy, 7.1 fl oz / 220 ml

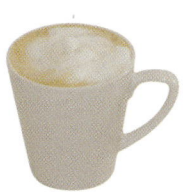

Hot milk drink, 6.7 fl oz / 200 ml

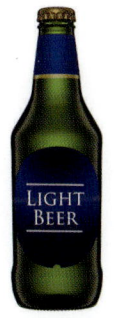

Beer, stubbie light, 12.5 fl oz / 375 ml

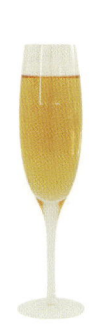

Sparkling wine, 5 fl oz / 150 ml

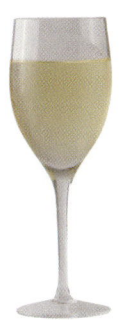

White wine, 5 fl oz / 150 ml

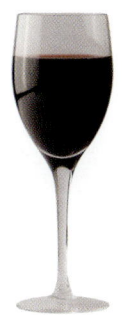

Red wine, 5 fl oz / 150 ml

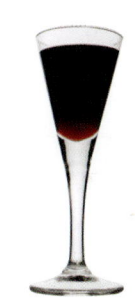

Liqueur, most varieties, 2 fl oz / 60 ml

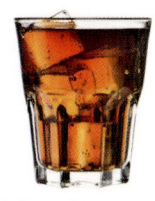

Spirit and diet mixer, most varieties, 1.5 fl oz / 45 ml spirit + 5 fl oz / 150 ml mixer

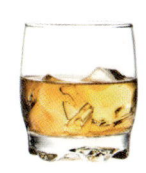

Spirits, most varieties, 1.5 fl oz / 45 ml

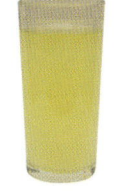

Soft drink, 6.7 fl oz / 200 ml

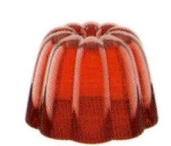

Jelly, with sugar, ¾ cup

Add your own favourite Add On serves to this list by referring to Allan Borushek's *The CalorieKing Calorie Fat and Carbohydrate Counter* or apps CalorieKing or My Fitness Pal. Calculate a serve size which contains approximately **100 Calories** / 420 kJ.

APPENDIX | 133

appendix 3

free foods = <20 Calories / 85 kJ

'Free foods' refer to foods that are very low in Calories, contributing 20 Calories / 85 kJ or less in a typical serve. It is safe to add one of these in the amount shown to any meal. Water and mineral water can be added freely, and you can consider a cupful of salad or free vegetables as a 'free food' serve.

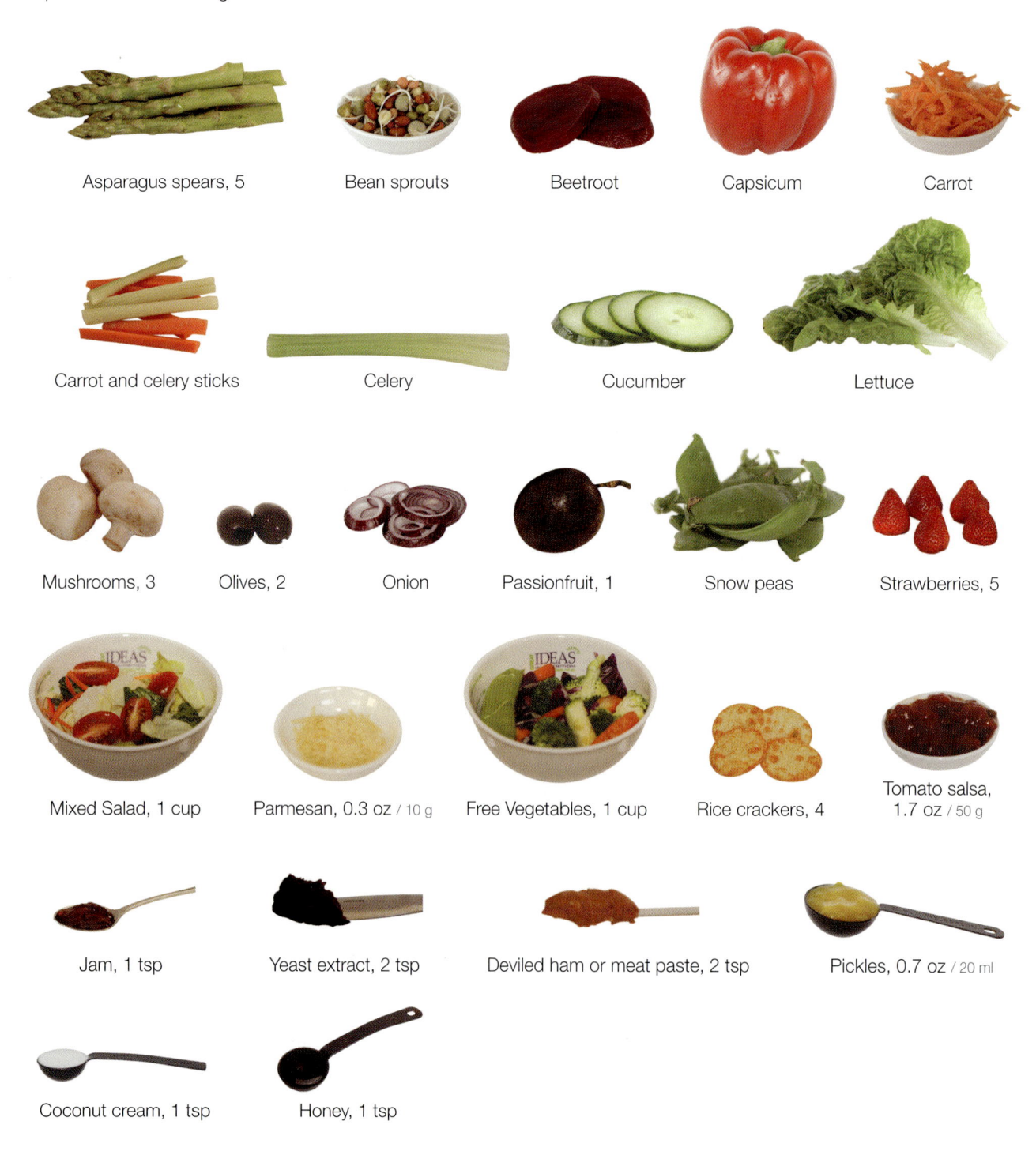

- Asparagus spears, 5
- Bean sprouts
- Beetroot
- Capsicum
- Carrot
- Carrot and celery sticks
- Celery
- Cucumber
- Lettuce
- Mushrooms, 3
- Olives, 2
- Onion
- Passionfruit, 1
- Snow peas
- Strawberries, 5
- Mixed Salad, 1 cup
- Parmesan, 0.3 oz / 10 g
- Free Vegetables, 1 cup
- Rice crackers, 4
- Tomato salsa, 1.7 oz / 50 g
- Jam, 1 tsp
- Yeast extract, 2 tsp
- Deviled ham or meat paste, 2 tsp
- Pickles, 0.7 oz / 20 ml
- Coconut cream, 1 tsp
- Honey, 1 tsp

appendix 3
free foods *continued*

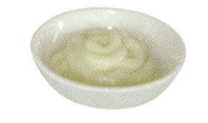

Mayonnaise, fat free, 0.7 oz / 20 g

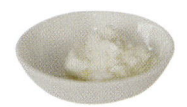

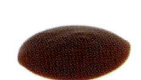

Sour cream, 1 tsp

Low fat sauce (eg tomato) 0.7 oz / 20 ml

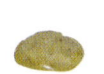

High fat sauce (eg bearnaise), 1 tsp

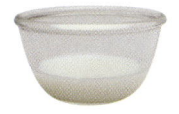

Milk, all types, 1 fl oz / 30 ml

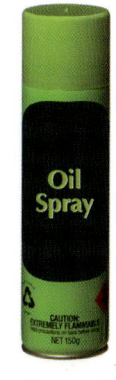

Spray oil (2 second spray)

Sugar, 1 cube

Chocolate, 1 square

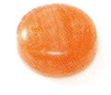

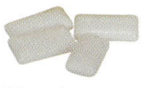

Cough lolly, 1

Chewing gum, all types, 4 pieces

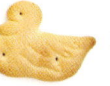

Animal crackers, 2

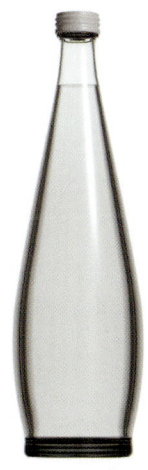

Water or mineral water (any time)

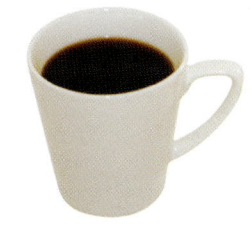

Black herbal tea or coffee with 1 tsp sugar or 1 fl oz / 30 ml milk

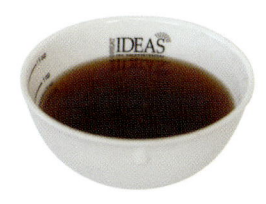

Consomme / broth / stock, 1 cup

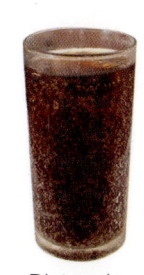

Diet soda, 8 fl oz / 250 ml

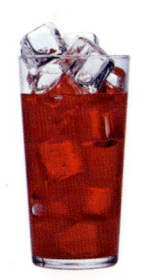

Diet Cordial, prepared, 8 fl oz / 250 ml

Add your own favourite free food serves to this list by referring to Allan Borushek's *The CalorieKing Calorie Fat and Carbohydrate Counter* **or apps CalorieKing or My Fitness Pal. Calculate a serve size which contains approximately 20 Calories** / 85 kJ **or less.**

APPENDIX | 135

appendix 4

My meal plan

Breakfast

Morning snack

Lunch

Afternoon snack

Dinner

Supper snack

appendix 4
My meal plan

Breakfast

Morning snack

Lunch

Afternoon snack

Dinner

Supper snack

appendix 5

menu planner

Use this planner to plan your week's food intake. Put all the ingredients for the meals straight onto the shopping list so you have every single herb and spice to make the meals perfect.

	BREAKFAST	LUNCH	DINNER	SNACKS
MONDAY				
TUESDAY				
WEDNESDAY				
THURSDAY				
FRIDAY				
SATURDAY				
SUNDAY				

appendix 5
shopping list

Groceries

Meat, seafood and poultry

Fruit & Vegetables

Dairy

Other

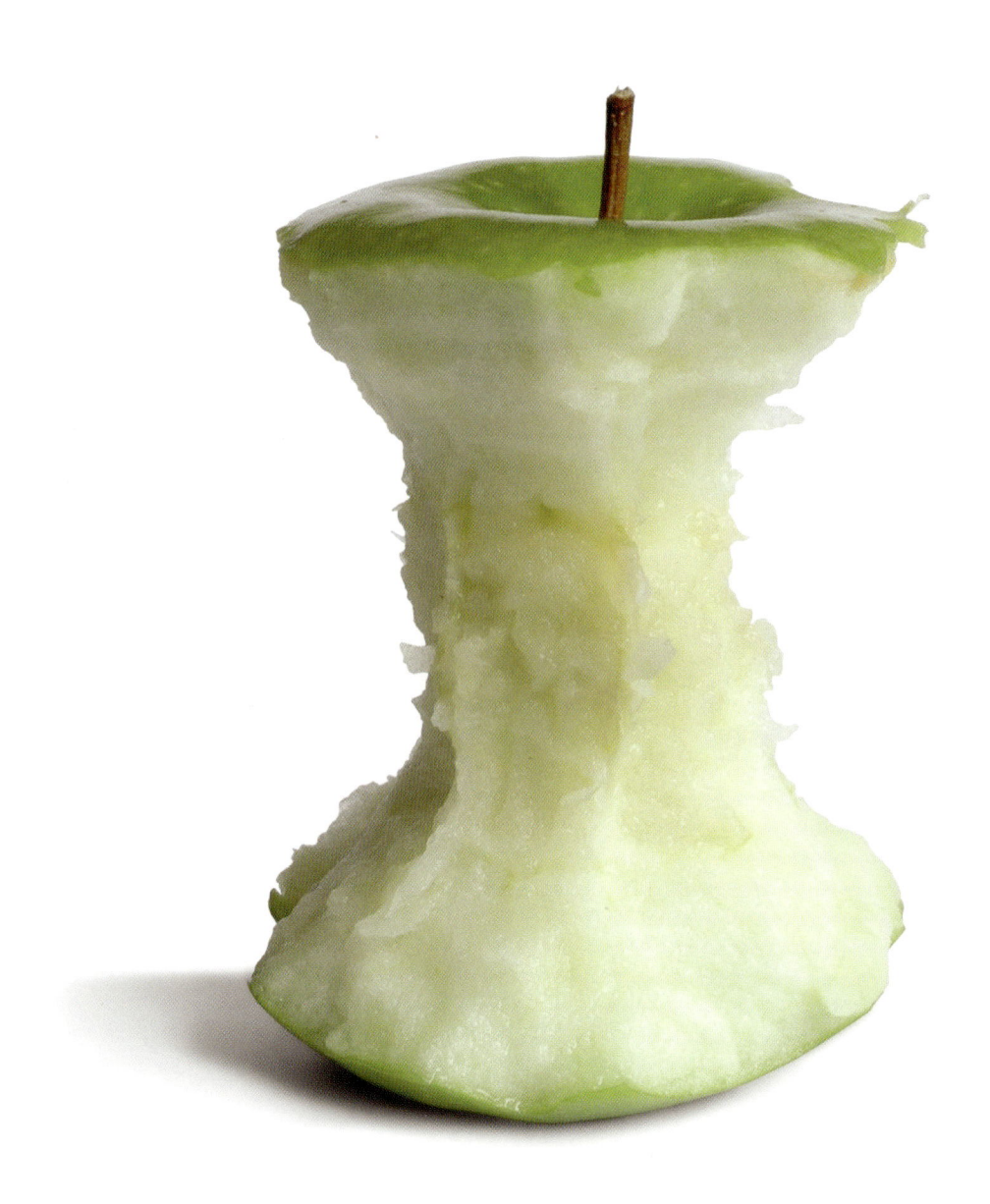

A final word…

I think legislation should be introduced that requires that the information on the nutrition panel relates to a realistic serving size.

I think there needs to be support for companies who package foods in serving sizes that match Calorie needs.

I'd like to see the 'party food' section of the supermarket move into a separate shop so that we are making a conscious decision to go and purchase these foods, rather than having them leap into our trolleys while doing the groceries. I think if we only actually ate cakes and lollies and chips and drank soft drink and alcohol at parties, we wouldn't be in this mess. Instead we're led to believe that a king sized chocolate bar is an acceptable purchase while filling up with petrol. In fact the attendants suggestive-sell chocolate bars in some service stations.

I'm pleased to see the Calorie contents displayed in food outlets because data from New York proves that when you see that the muffin you like to eat with your coffee contains 500 or 600 Calories 2100 or 2520 kJ it is less appealing, resulting in an average decrease in calorie intake by 6% for every purchase made.

Come and join us on facebook to let us know how you're going and hear about new products as they become available, www.facebook.com/portionperfection.

Portion Perfection Products

The purple version of Portion Perfection contains plans for men, women and children and a larger plate than the bariatric version. The bowls, snack bible and hypnotherapy apply to everyone.

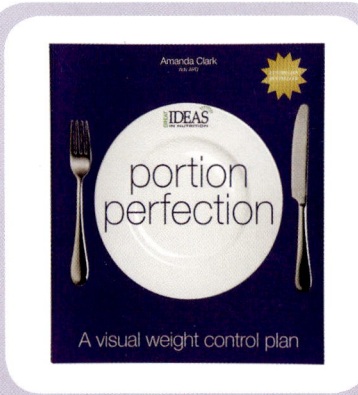

**Portion Perfection -
A visual weight control plan**
– Printed or Electronic versions

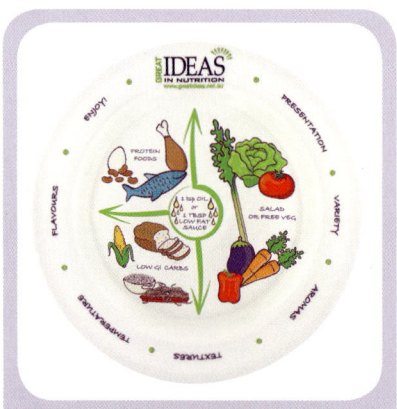

**Portion Perfection Plate
in Porcelain or Melamine**
(Porcelain currently only available in Australia)

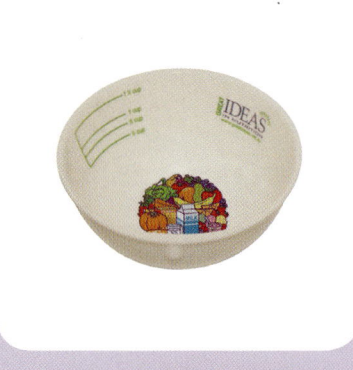

**Portion Perfection Bowl
in Porcelain or Melamine**
(Porcelain currently only available in Australia)

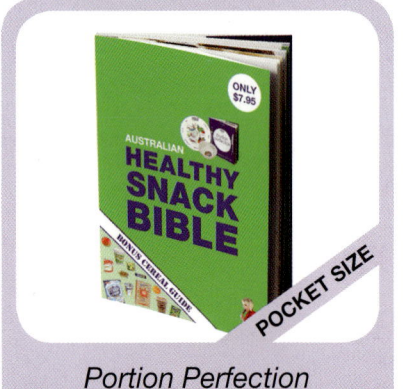

**Portion Perfection
Healthy Snack Bible**
– US and UK versions coming soon

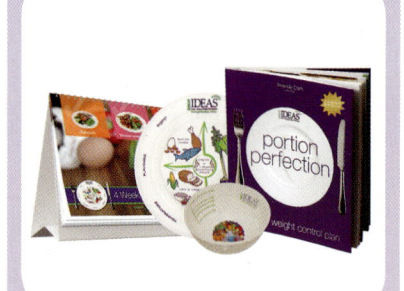

Portion Perfection Pack
– Special price

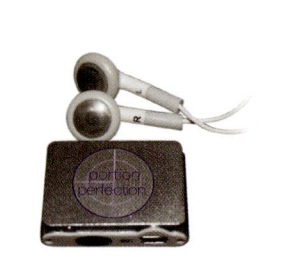

**Hypnotherapy Mp3 player
or direct file download**
(Player currently only available in Australia)

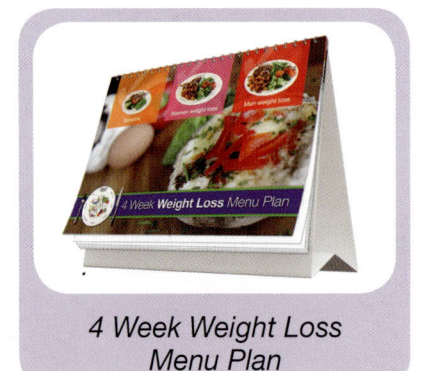

**4 Week Weight Loss
Menu Plan**

Join Portion Perfection on facebook for updates on healthy products.

Bariatric Products

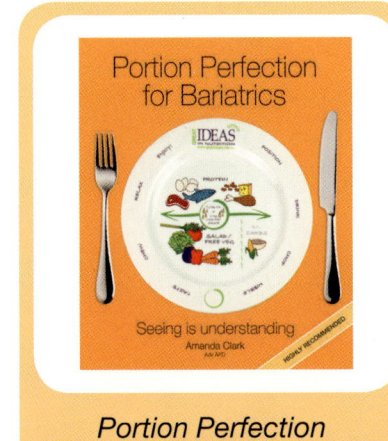

Portion Perfection for Bariatrics
– Printed or Electronic versions

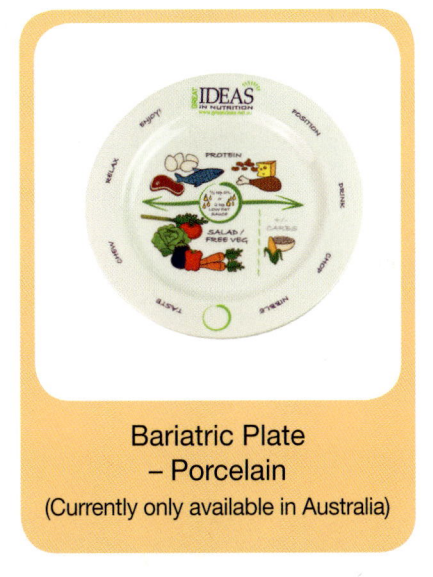

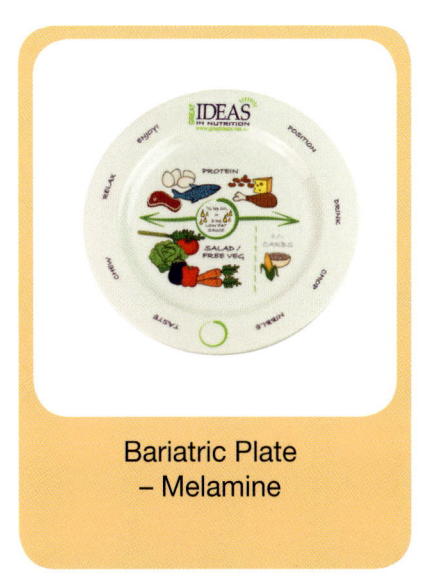

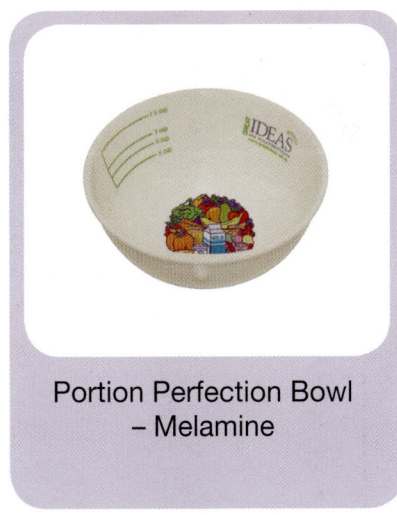

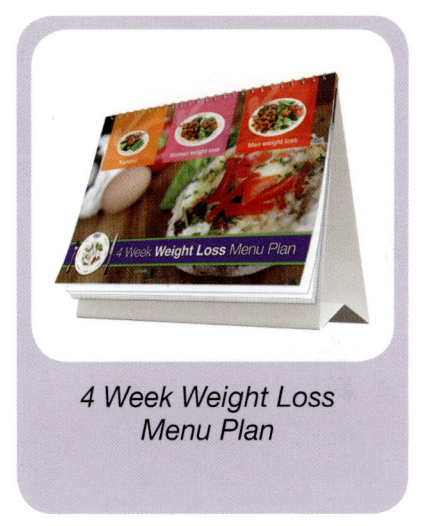

Bariatric Plate – Porcelain
(Currently only available in Australia)

Bariatric Plate – Melamine

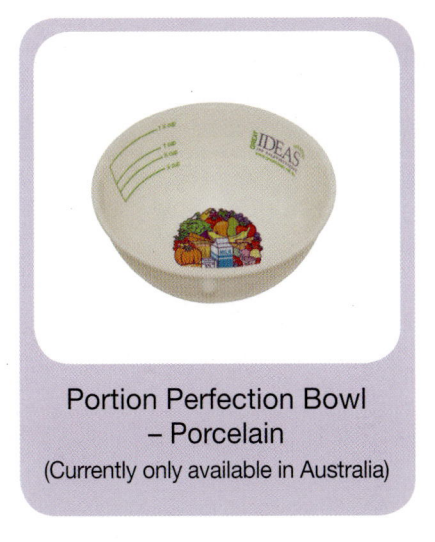

Portion Perfection Bowl – Porcelain
(Currently only available in Australia)

Portion Perfection Bowl – Melamine

4 Week Weight Loss Menu Plan

Bariatric Pack – Special price

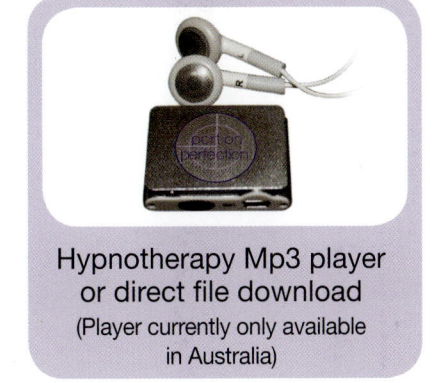

Hypnotherapy Mp3 player or direct file download
(Player currently only available in Australia)

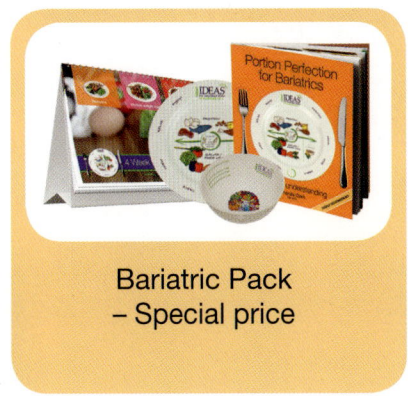

Visit our international website
www.portiondiet.com
for the best healthy lifestyle resources available.

enjoy!